SHRED IT!

Robert Cheeke

"Robert Cheeke is one of the most influential vegan athletes of all time. He is the most recognizable vegan bodybuilder in the world and has also made a name for himself as an inspirational speaker and fitness motivator. As the first to publish a book on vegan bodybuilding and create an extremely popular website on the same topic, Robert pioneered a movement. Now, he takes it to the next level (I would expect nothing less from him) with this new book that speaks to everyone, at every level of fitness and health and gives the reader the tools to improve their life in many important ways. This is a MUST READ for anyone who wants to be fit, strong, and healthy."

— **Brenda Carey,**
Editor in Chief/Founder, *Vegan Health & Fitness Magazine*

"Robert Cheeke is living proof that you can get ripped while fueling yourself with delicious plant-based foods. So many athletes are now tapping into the power of leaving animals off their plates, and Robert was a pioneer in this field. Whether you want to be an elite athlete or just want to shed some fat, get *Shred It!* to learn how to achieve your goals, and thrive while doing it."

— **Paul Shapiro, The Humane Society of the United States**

"I can personally say that through all of my vigorous training and competing over the years, plant-based meals have left me feeling the best on a daily basis. I feel as if I perform at a much higher level, more consistently, and I just simply feel better. Though I am not 100 percent vegan, I believe this book has beneficial information that anyone and everyone can use. Robert does a phenomenal job providing facts and information along with encouraging and motivating messages about nutrition and fitness. Anyone, from a professional athlete to someone simply seeking a healthier lifestyle, can take something away from this that will positively affect their life and bring them closer to achieving their goals."

— **Dan Molls, NFL Linebacker**

"Since 2009, I endorsed and adopted Robert Cheeke's plant-based diet. Now I practice and share his vegan lifestyle dietary suggestions and I've never felt better. *Shred It!* is the bible for the perfect healthy vegan lifestyle that will answer all your questions along the way and help you achieve your goals!"

— **Georges Laraque,**
former 13-year National Hockey League (NHL) veteran

"Robert Cheeke does it again. Yet another great, easy-to-read reference full of useful information that anyone from plant-based veterans, to those who are simply veg-curious can happily sink their teeth into. A definite future-classic in the Vegan library."

— **Mac Danzig, Ultimate Fighting Champion**

"This is great and it's about time someone has produced an insightful, detailed book that relates to true health and fitness and how to fuel that process. Robert Cheeke has written that book and I feel safe and secure sending all of the people that always ask me questions such as, 'Where do you get your protein?' and 'Will I wither away?' directly to *Shred It!*. Thanks, Robert."

— **Phil Collen, co-lead guitarist of Def Leppard**

"Who says you can't be strong, buff, and healthy on a plant-based diet? Robert Cheeke shows you exactly how to do just that in this helpful book. He has years of experience and knows what he is talking about. So pick up this book and listen!"

— **Emily Deschanel, actress, star of the hit TV show, *Bones***

"Robert Cheeke is a champion bodybuilder who has excelled. In *Shred It!*, he explains how to burn fat and build muscle following a delicious, healthy plant-based diet. Whether you are looking to tone up or bulk up, this book will help you get shredded!"

— **Gene Baur, President of Farm Sanctuary**

"Robert Cheeke illuminates the athletic world with a huge reality check in *Shred It!*, making it impossible not to be infused with inspiration. Combining effective tips, tools, and advice founded in research and experience along with encouragement to tap into your true motivation and goals, Cheeke debunks the pervasive nutrition myths and empowers you on your road to optimal fitness. *Shred It!* puts to rest the argument that plants can't power ultimate athletic achievement."

— **Julieanna Hever, MS, RD, CPT,**
author of *The Complete Idiot's Guide to Plant-Based Nutrition,*
The Vegiterranean Diet*, and host of *What Would Julieanna Do?

"Robert Cheeke knows how to sculpt a body and in *Shred It!*, he shares this knowledge with the rest of us—not just aspiring bodybuilders, but regular folks who want to look terrific, feel good about themselves, and get genuinely healthy in the bargain. And he's written this book like a supportive friend or dedicated coach—a really great guy to have in your corner."

— **Victoria Moran, author of *Main Street Vegan***

"Robert breaks it all down for us in easy to digest pieces of information and inspiration to help us build the bodies we desire fueled on plant-based nutrition! Robert is one competitive bodybuilder who I trust for fat loss and muscle mass building protocol. Let's *Shred It!*"

— **Ani Phyo, wellness expert, best-selling author,**
and founder of AniPhyo.com

"*Shred It!* by Robert Cheeke is a must read for anybody who wants to learn the truth behind the foods we eat and their relationship to a healthy and fit body, mind, and soul. Nothing is as powerful as understanding how our body works and knowing the what, when, why, and how behind feeding our body to get the results we desire. Robert has spent decades experimenting and learning these keys and has kindly passed that journey's knowledge onto us. In a world where meat, eggs, and dairy are perceived as king; at a time when the health and fitness industry is full of propaganda, misinformation, and outright lies, Robert sheds a bright light on how anybody can 'Shred It' with a smart whole-food, plant-based diet. Whether omnivore or herbivore, novice or professional athlete like myself, everybody can gain great new insight from Robert Cheeke's *Shred It!*"

— **Austin Aries, plant-based, multi-time World Champion Professional Wrestler**

"Whether you're looking to build muscle or just trying to eat better, Robert Cheeke has you covered with *Shred It!* In the gym, he shows how to set realistic and achievable goals, while offering encouragement that will help avoid setbacks and common mistakes. Then he maps out a workout plan to help you build muscle and strengthen our core.

"At the table, he shreds misperceptions about plant-based nutrition, showing how to maximize carbohydrates and protein for optimal energy and strength, and offers easy-to-follow meal plans that won't bore your palate.

"Finally, Robert takes you to the kitchen with a fun collection of 50 soups, salads, and hearty dishes made out of whole foods—no phony-baloney faux meats here! Best of all, these healthy recipes are fun to make and designed to help you reach your fitness goals. Who would have guessed that getting shredded would taste this good?"

— **Grant Butler, Food Writer, *The Oregonian***

"Robert Cheeke exemplifies how eating a plant-based diet, having a compassion-filled outlook, and leading a motion-filled lifestyle contributes to amazing health results. His eagerly awaited book *Shred It!* shares important information, practical tips, and incredible inspiration that's sure to motivate and delight readers and fans."

— **John Pierre, author of *The Pillars of Health*, and founder of johnpierre.com**

"Plant-based eating is on the cutting edge, with more athletes discovering it every day. Now, Robert Cheeke has created the perfect introduction for reaching one's athletic potential on a plant-based diet. This book is what many of us have been waiting for, and what anyone who cares about their health and fitness cannot afford to miss."

— Mark Devries, Director and Producer of *Speciesism: The Movie*

"A must-read for any health-conscious person. Robert Cheeke has done his homework so you can get educated as well as motivated by his wise and inspiring messages."

— George Eisman, MA, MS, RD (Registered Dietitian)
Nutrition Director, Coalition for Cancer Prevention

"*Shred It!* has everything you need to know to lose weight now! With Robert's simple plan you can burn that extra fat and gain muscle all while eating Robert's whole-foods recipes that are easy to prepare and taste incredible. Say good-bye to hunger and say hello to a new lean, toned, and energized YOU!"

— Chloe Coscarelli, cookbook author

"As soon as you become vegan, your friends, relatives, and peers force you to become something of a nutrition expert. But you can go your whole life not knowing the best way to exercise to get ripped. Robert breaks it down here in such an easy, accessible way. With sample workouts and menu plans, he takes the guesswork out of achieving the healthy body you want. The athletes whose stories he tells and whose jaw-dropping physical transformations he features will inspire you to get off your tush and shred it—for your health, for animals, and for the planet."

— Marisa Miller Wolfson, Creator and Executive Producer
of the award-winning film, *Vegucated*

"Robert Cheeke clearly knows his stuff when it comes to whole-food, plant-based nutrition, and understands exactly what it takes to add muscle and burn fat. But in *Shred It!*, he goes beyond the physical, challenging us to take our mental games to the next level—by setting goals, making real commitments, creating accountability, walking the walk to embody the qualities we value."

— Matt Frazier, vegan ultramarathoner,
author of *No Meat Athlete*, and founder of nomeatathlete.com

"What Robert has done with this book and his overall dedication to the plant-based lifestyle, has been inspiring to myself and other vegans, breaking through myths about what's required to be both vegan and physically strong enough to compete at bodybuilding's elite levels."

— **Daniel Negreanu, professional poker player,**
2013 WSOP Player of the Year

"Robert lays the foundation of health and fitness with a clear and effective method to achieve popular fitness goals, burn fat, and build muscle . . . the healthy way that will not only cause your body to look good, but also to reach optimal long-term health. Something most other fitness approaches fail to do."

— **Elizabeth Kucinich, Policy Director, Center for Food Safety**

"A thorough and comprehensive review of bodybuilding principles and theory from a vegan perspective. Overall, an excellent read."

— **Milton Mills, M.D.**

SHRED IT!

By Robert Cheeke

Gaven Press
Los Angeles, CA

Cover Design: Jody Conners and Richard Watts
Page Layout: Jody Conners
Front Cover photography: Brenda Carey
Editing: Karen Reddick

www.veganbodybuilding.com

Gaven Press
Los Angeles, CA

ISBN 978-0-9843916-1-5

Printed and bound in the United States of America
by Maverick Publications • Bend, Oregon

Definitions

Shred: To burn body fat and tone one's body into a fit and lean physique.

Shredded: The result of reducing one's body fat while building muscle, creating a lean, toned and muscular physique.

> **Example:** He trained in the gym five days a week and after a few months he was shredded!

Vegan: "The word 'veganism' denotes a philosophy and way of living which seeks to exclude—as far as is possible and practical—all forms of exploitation of, and cruelty to, animals for food, clothing or any other purpose; and by extension, promotes the development and use of animal-free alternatives for the benefit of humans, animals and the environment. In dietary terms it denotes the practice of dispensing with all products derived wholly or partly from animals."

— Donald Watson, vegan activist who coined the term "vegan" in 1944

Whole-food, plant-based diet: "A plant-based diet emphasizes vegetables, fruits, legumes, and whole grains. These foods are good sources of protein, carbohydrates, fat, vitamins, and minerals. They are also naturally lower in calories than foods made from animals. Colorful plant foods are also good sources of *phytochemicals*. Phytochemicals are naturally present in plant foods, and they can help to protect our body's cells from damage by cancer-causing agents. They also help support overall health."

Source: http://shrp.rutgers.edu/dept/nutr/INI/
health/documents/Plant-BasedDiet.pdf

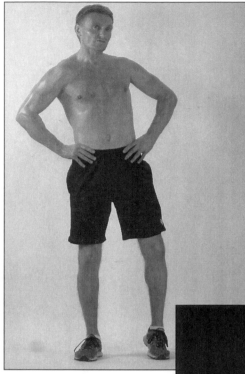

*Robert Cheeke - January 2013,
following a six-month break
from weight training*

*Robert Cheeke - April 2013,
73 days after
returning to training.
Photo by Melissa Schwartz
theveganrevolution.net*

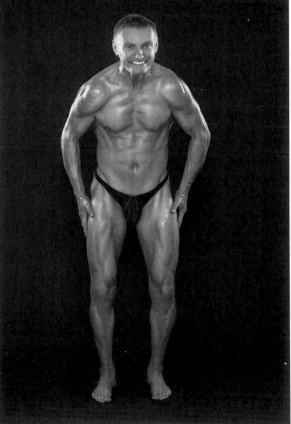

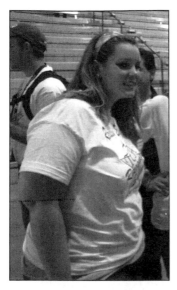

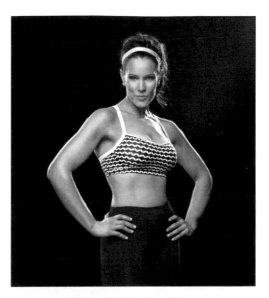

Tricia Kelly - 2009, before a
plant-based diet

Tricia Kelly - 2013, after 3.5 years on
a plant-based diet
Photo by Melissa Schwartz - theveganrevolution.net

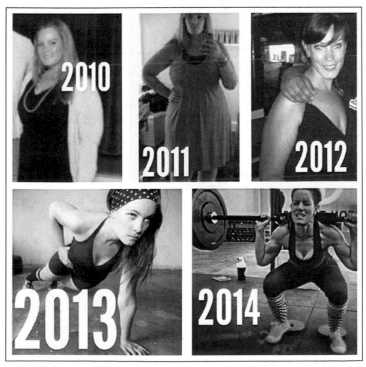

Tricia Kelly through the years of her transformation

GET SHREDDED!

Disclaimer

The contents of this book have not been approved by the FDA or any other governing body concerning the nutrition and fitness advice and suggestions provided within. Though the author is certified in plant-based nutrition, and numerous nutritionists, doctors, and experts have reviewed and endorsed *Shred It!*, you are advised to consult your physician or your own nutrition expert before adopting the programs outlined in this book.

The information, including meal plans and exercises, are recommendations to be used as guidelines and models. Consult your doctor, trainer, or nutritionist before embarking on one of the programs described in this book.

The author, editor, publisher, printer, contributors and others involved in this publication release themselves from any liability involving injury or loss as a result of applying the recommendations within this book.

Above all else, use reason and common sense when applying principles outlined in *Shred It!*, pursue meaningful goals, and aim to be healthy and happy.

Table of Contents

Robert Cheeke

To the less fortunate human and nonhuman animals
I am committed to helping.
You have value, you are appreciated, and you are loved.
May you be happy, may you be at ease,
and may you be free from suffering.

Introduction

"Motivation is what gets you started. Habit is what keeps you going."
— Jim Ryun

When I was a young boy, while my mother shopped at the local Safeway grocery store, I would pass the time hanging out in the magazine section. As I took a break from looking at baseball card and video game magazines, I looked at the covers of muscle magazines that adorned the shelves and wondered, *How do they do it?*

Two decades later I would walk into grocery stores and see myself on the covers of muscle magazines and realize that I had sufficiently satisfied my childhood inquisitive mind. I had answered my own questions through a combination of setting clear goals, working harder than most are willing to work, and from being consistent, accountable, and transparent about who and what I wanted to be when I grew up. I decided not to let perceived limitations keep me from achieving what I wanted to accomplish. It didn't matter that I did not have ideal genetics, or a lot of money, or famous friends. I knew where I was headed and I propelled myself there via the most over-used cliché I can think of right now, through blood, sweat, and tears (though not necessarily in that order). I'd say more sweat than anything, and quite a few tears, especially on leg training day or during moments when I realized childhood dreams coming true.

Over the past two decades that I have been a plant-based athlete, I have fielded countless questions about two common themes in health and fitness. Aside from questions regarding where I find adequate amounts of the seemingly elusive nutrient—protein—the most common questions asked are how to effectively burn fat and build muscle. If you think about it, most of us desire at least one of these objectives. Essentially everyone has some sort of health or fitness goal. We all want to lose weight, reduce body fat, build muscle, have more energy, or some other desired result we claim to care about, because we believe it will enhance our life.

Burning fat is a common objective shared by the majority of the population, but amazingly, most people don't have a clue how to properly achieve fat loss. Likewise, there are plenty of skinny people wanting to get bigger and stronger but feel that it is not in the cards for them, that they don't have the right genetics, and assume it just isn't meant to be. That perspective often results from not having learned how to properly achieve their goals, and from giving up far too early in their pursuit. These common misunderstandings about health and fitness, related to one's ability to achieve goals, compelled me to write this book. I have been down these roads many times and my experiences will help you avoid pitfalls, will give you the motivation you need to achieve your fitness goals, and perhaps will help land you on the cover of an idealistic news media publication someday.

Everybody claims to have goals, yet statistically, very few people achieve them on a regular basis. Whether it is shredding up or bulking up, we all have a desire to change. The principles I will share with you can be life changing and give you the fundamental tools to take action and make your health and fitness dreams happen. Not only will I show you how to burn fat and build muscle effectively in ways that will work for you, I will teach you how to set goals, create action plans, and achieve desired results that will benefit you beyond the weight room and sports field.

As a skinny 120-pound teenager who adopted a plant-based diet and vegan lifestyle in the mid-1990s and went on to be a two-time champion bodybuilder, weighing nearly 200 pounds, I have first-hand experience in building my body and then shredding it down to get ripped for the body-building stage. Today, I am at a point where I understand the science and the process of changing my physique so well, I can literally sculpt my body into any shape I want. I know the formulas from years of trial and error, and successes and failures. Though it is true that each of our bodies are slightly different in how they process nutrients and metabolize fats, and we all have different genetics and caloric intake needs based on numerous factors, there are general, but also specific, approaches that work for most of us. In this book I am going to show you precisely how to effectively shred fat and bulk up with quality muscle, all on a whole-food, plant-based diet, and vegan lifestyle.

You will learn the following important steps toward achieving your health and fitness goals:

- How to properly set achievable goals.

- How to create a consistent action plan.

- Recognizing the #1 mistake people make when trying to lose weight.

- Understanding what could be holding you back.

- How to overcome obstacles and setbacks and maintain a positive outlook.

- How to succeed in the fat loss and muscle building pursuit once and for all.

You will learn the three most effective methods of burning fat, and a tried and true formula for building muscle. You will read inspiring case studies, transformation stories, and see real results from those who have dramatically changed their physiques (and their lives) in the ways that you are striving to achieve as well.

A plant-based diet happens to be an incredibly healthy and efficient way to eat to fuel the health and fitness goals many of us share. A compassionate vegan lifestyle (abstaining from the consumption or use of animal products in food and clothing, while avoiding products tested on animals and rejecting entities that confine and harm animals) is perfectly aligned with eating plant-based whole foods and living a healthy life. There are many compelling reasons to follow a plant-based diet and vegan lifestyle. Here are ten:

1. Best diet to prevent and even reverse disease.

2. Diet and lifestyle that yields the most energy.

3. Best diet to aid in recovery after exercise.

4. Fiber is only found in plants and is of paramount health importance.

5. Cholesterol is only found in animal products and should be avoided.

6. Plants provide the optimal sources of nutrition in their original form.

7. Most environmentally-friendly diet.

8. Nobody has to be raised on a factory farm and slaughtered for you to eat.

9. Least amount of resources used to produce food to feed the masses.

10. The most compassionate diet and lifestyle one can follow.

After reading this book, you will know how to sculpt your body into nearly any shape you want, will have a better understanding of the relationship between goal setting and attainment, and you will be equipped with the formulas and tools to build your own desired physique. I am confident this book will change the way you look at health, fitness, food, and setting goals, and will inspire you to set your sights high for a bright future ahead. When you discover the inherent value and merit in making health and fitness a true priority, and grant it credence, as a consistent truth revealed through your actions, you will no doubt become a role model to many and could quite possibly discover your happiest self.

Are you ready to get shredded? There is no better time than *right now* to pursue meaningful and worthwhile goals. Follow *your* passion and make it happen!

– CHAPTER 1 –

Getting Started –
Are You Ready to Get Shredded?

> *"It is good to have an end to journey toward;*
> *but it is the journey that matters, in the end."*
>
> — Ernest Hemingway

Would having a better understanding of how your body burns fat and builds muscle help you in your health and athletic pursuits? Sure it would. It helps millions of athletes every day. Why not you? Knowledge of how your body works is a key to enhancing athletic performance. As athletes, this is what we seek. What works for athletes, works for the rest of us too, even if we don't consider ourselves to be particularly physically fit. That is the beauty of proven health and fitness principles, they work rather effectively when we follow the rules closely with consistency and accountability. Let's learn how to most efficiently get from point A to point E in pursuit of our goals, in order to have a clearer vision of how to attain them. Understanding the roles that points B, C, and D play in reaching our goals can be the difference between success and failure. These are the points that will reveal our strengths and weaknesses by showing us precisely where we took the right, or wrong, turns. Mistakes are important teaching tools if we remain open to learning from them. Success and failure in athletics teach valuable lessons that can carry over to other areas of life too.

When I give lectures throughout North America, I often ask audiences if they have ever wanted to lose five or ten pounds or reduce body fat. Almost everyone raises their hand. My follow-up question asks the audience if they know how to get into an effective fat-burning zone to actually burn fat and lose weight. There are very few hands raised at this point, if any at all. If we claim to want to be able to burn fat, yet we do not know how to do it, how can we really expect to achieve it? It is no wonder millions of people are confused, discouraged, frustrated, and often give up on their fitness goals because they simply do not see results. And who can blame them? It takes a strong-willed person to keep going when results are not coming in. When the desire to change is there but the outcome does not reflect the effort, there is some other issue at play; namely, a misunderstanding of how the process works. Trying to burn fat or build muscle without knowing how the processes work is like trying to prepare a meal without knowing the ingredients to the recipe. It is not going to turn out the way it looks in the book, or taste like the properly made end result. Exercise results count on systematic actions that lead to desired outcomes, just as learning how to speak a new language or learning any new skill requires a specific and proper approach. If you do not study attentively and consistently and practice regularly, you will not learn a new language, just as you will not burn fat or build muscle effectively unless you know how those processes work and apply appropriate action.

If you are tired of hitting roadblocks, are losing patience with plateaus, and want to make some real progress, you should take the time to understand how your body produces energy, burns fuel, and repairs muscle tissue. From what fuel to consume, to how to get into that elusive fat-burning zone, to which approaches will truly build muscle, gain strength, or improve endurance, knowing is certainly half the battle. If knowing is half the battle, doing is the other half. What you do with the information you learn is up to you. What actions can you take to improve upon today to be better tomorrow?

Answer the following questions as honestly as you can. Why is your health and fitness important to you? Who cares about health anyway? Who cares about fitness? In fact, who cares about the animals and the environment? If you do, state your case. If you can't find meaning in health and fitness and find value in its pursuit, you won't achieve your goals. The reason you won't succeed if you don't care about your health and fitness is because it is really hard to be disciplined, dedicated, and committed to health and fitness when you'd rather be doing something else. The easiest thing in the world is to give up, and far too many people do it far too often in too many areas of life, including fitness. Did you know that the most common day people give up on New Year's Resolutions is January 17? Most of us set seemingly meaningful goals and after two and a half weeks determine the effort was just too much and postpone any future endeavors in health and fitness for another year. This is a cycle that many people will go through their entire lives, never reaching their destination. It doesn't have to be this way, and I have some solutions to help make January 17 just another day on the calendar in which you actively pursue your goals.

Many people would rather do anything than eat healthy foods and exercise regularly. By "do anything," I mean watch television, eat junk food, aimlessly surf the Internet, and similar counterproductive actions that occupy the majority of our free time. These behaviors will not support your health and fitness goals and are some of the primary obstacles holding people back, keeping countless individuals complacent. Distractions become excuses and excuses attempt to wipe our hands clean of responsibility and accountability. Removing ownership of responsibility attempts to justify our shortcomings and seeks to blame anything or anyone but ourselves for undesired outcomes. Today is the day you decide to own up to your actions and strive for success. I'm happy to be part of your journey, supporting your efforts as you seek your personal best.

To set yourself up to be successful, you have to be able to answer the fundamental questions stated above: What does health and fitness mean to you? How bad do you want it? What are you willing to do to make it happen? Do you *wish* for a better health outcome and a fitter body someday, or are you ready to start *working* toward it today, not even waiting until tomorrow, but literally starting right now? Show your enthusiasm to set higher standards, building a stronger body and mind inside and out. Drop to the floor and pump out some push-ups to demonstrate your level of commitment to the new you. How many did you just do? Those who find it within themselves to rise up and accept the challenge to replace who they are now, with who they can become, will indeed succeed and achieve.

Everyone talks about getting healthier, losing weight, building muscle, or some other health objective, but very few actually achieve it. Why is this the case, and how can you avoid being a statistic as part of the norm? Here's the key: Strive to be anything but average. Average does the bare minimum, average attains mediocre results, and average sets the bar just high enough to get by. Make it a point to be remarkable in health and fitness. When you are remarkable, you helplessly inspire others because you confidently lead by example and your actions speak for themselves. If being average is something you're currently content with, I have a challenge for you. Visualize your best self, right now. What does it look like? What does it feel like? What health and fitness dreams do you aim to achieve? Take a moment to visualize what this remarkable state of health feels like when you engage your senses to focus on this vision. If there is a formula to make this outcome a reality, why do so many people struggle to achieve happiness in these incredibly important areas of life?

The problem is that we're too distracted with other aspects of our lives that dominate our time. We all have 1,440 minutes each day to do as we wish, and unfortunately for most of us, exercise and healthy lifestyle decisions get left out and pushed to the back burner. Consider this: The world is full of people who are lying to themselves and others about what they really care about. If you say that your passion is skiing but you live in the desert, you're not being honest. If you really loved skiing you would move from the desert to the mountains. If you claim to love the outdoors but spend all day in a cubicle, you don't *really* love the outdoors. There are plenty of ways to live and work outside if it really tugs at your heart. Don't let life pass you by because you're doing things you're not passionate about. If you really love something you'll find a way to make it happen. This has been one of the truest and purest realizations I have come to in all my years exploring the relationship between high levels of health and fitness and their influence on happiness. The reality is, too many people love television, smart phones, and social networking way too much, and they don't love their own bodies or themselves enough to make healthy decisions day in and day out. That may be hard to hear, but it's true. Nothing reveals our true priorities like our actions. You may say your priority is to go to the gym, but in reality your priority is posting witty status updates and waiting for pats on the back in the form of "likes" and comments while watching TV to pass the time. You may say your priority is to eat whole foods, but the reality is that your friends like eating pizza and ice cream and you'd rather participate in that activity than the healthy one you outlined and posted about publicly online. We've all been there. We've been fooling ourselves about what our real priorities are, but as soon as you become totally transparent with your actions, you can be held accountable and you can make better decisions that support the goals you truly care about. Simply acknowledging some of your current behavior in relation to the impact it has on your health, and evaluating it as objectively as possible, puts you in a powerful position to make personal change. I applaud you for taking your health seriously, because you are no doubt a role model to many and you have a wonderful opportunity to positively influence those around you. I value your commitment to becoming your personal best. You really can make your goals a reality, and it starts with making them a true priority. When you believe in yourself wholeheartedly, others will believe in you too.

Here's the first step: Do yourself a favor and be honest as often as possible. Even when nobody is watching or holding you accountable, don't stop short of your tenth repetition in the gym, or settle for fifteen push-ups when you know you can do twenty. Don't pull up a quarter mile short of your planned mileage when you're on a run by yourself. Don't stop your hour-long workout at the fifty-seven-minute mark. Conversely, notice what happens when you do an eleventh rep, twenty-one push-ups, run a quarter mile longer, or add another five minutes to your workout. If cutting corners has left you unfulfilled and hasn't helped you achieve your goals, what happens when you go above and beyond what you outlined for yourself? When you learn to hold yourself accountable and go the extra mile because you know it will pay dividends in the long run, contributing positively to your end result, you will expedite progress.

Transparency leads to accountability, which can lead to consistency, adaptation, and success. **This *is* the winning combination. Transparency + Accountability = Consistency, Adaptation, and Success.** You just have to want it badly enough. I can give you the nutrition and exercise tips to essentially guarantee success in your area of interest, but it doesn't mean a thing if you can't find it within yourself to make it a true priority in your life. If you can't find 40 minutes a day to exercise, because your 1,440 minutes each day are filled with other things that are unsupportive of your goals, then clearly we know what your priorities are. Evaluating real priorities can realistically estimate predictable outcomes. We all have busy lives, but the "I don't have time" explanation is no longer a valid excuse. At the end of the day, we choose what to do with our time. It is up to us to create time for healthy habits and to reduce time spent on unhealthy habits.

I'm here to help you get to the finish line to experience a new level of happiness. If other approaches haven't worked for you in the past, allow me to share the approach that has worked exceptionally well for me and many people I work with. I know what it takes to make physique transformations happen. I know what it takes to reclaim health and fitness through discipline and accountability. I know the pain of failing and suffering that comes from struggle, uncertainty, and confusion that is often associated with coming face to face with our own realities of where we are versus where we want to be. I know the rejuvenating feeling of picking myself up off the ground, promising myself I have much more to offer, convincing myself that my work ethic will reveal a different result next time. I understand what it feels like to be a beginner, to trespass beyond comfort zones, and challenge myself to improve.

The formula is easy. The willpower is the obstacle, and that lies in your hands. At the end of the day, the actual accountability is yours, and you live with the decisions you make and actions you do or do not take. What's it going to be? How much do you want to create a new you? Let's get shredded!

– CHAPTER 2 –

Setting Achievable Goals

> *"While intent is the seed of manifestation, action is the water that nourishes the seed. Your actions must reflect your goals in order to achieve true success."*
>
> — Steve Maraboli, *Life, the Truth and Being Free*

From my observations, perhaps the number one reason why people do not achieve their goals is because they did not set goals that were attainable. Their goals were too far out of reach, took too much work (at least more effort than they were willing to give), and became so daunting that the easiest thing was to just give up. Listen, I'm as much of a go-getter as it gets, and it pained me to write that opening sentence of this chapter. I wish that statement wasn't an assessment of my first-hand observations, and I wish that reality and outcome weren't the case. It saddens me to write about people setting lofty goals and not achieving them, but that's how it is. Somewhere along the way we got lost in a fantasy world of instant gratification and forgot about all the little steps along the way that lead to desired outcomes. We've lost patience in a fast-paced world and we're trying to go from point A to point E by cleverly bypassing points B, C, and D, without having to put in the hard work, but it doesn't always work that way.

When we disrespect the formulas, systems, and action steps on the road to achievement, we disrespect ourselves by not giving ourselves a real chance at success. We also disrespect others who follow the natural rules of nature, who have succeeded the old fashioned way by putting in the time, doing what it takes to elicit change and create results. I want people to aim high and go for it all, but it has to be within a certain context, given the prerequisite conditions to actually achieve lofty goals. Not everyone is an overachiever, a go-getter, or is one who inherently has what it takes to reach the highest levels of success. Some people have *it*, whatever *it* is, and you can sense this when you come across them. They shine and exude confidence and success in everything they do. Even if you don't think you have much of *it*, you can still succeed and achieve. Passion and hard work make up for a lack of talent, and skill can be learned over time. We have seen this play out in the lives of millions of people, who on the surface looked like they were plagued because of their body type, education, or poverty, but who rose above that because of their determination or charisma. I am a sincere fan of focusing on strengths and being the best we can, rather than focusing on bringing up weak areas to be more balanced, but I am also a fan of following your passion. If your passion and your strengths don't support one another, you can take either road: following your passion or your strength and in due time, you may find that they eventually meet up. This has been true for me in athletics and academics and other areas of life. Follow *either* your strengths *or* passions, and you will likely succeed because your strengths could become your passions and your passions pursued could become your strengths. If I had to choose one over the other, I would say follow your passions for personal fulfillment and follow your strengths for professional fulfillment, and whichever means the most is up to you.

Just as often as we set lofty goals that are a little out of reach, many of us underestimate our own capabilities and set goals that are not high enough. That's how a lot of our friends, family, and neighbors end up in complacent situations of contentment, but not happiness. Goals were set too low, were attained without a level of enthusiastic fulfillment, and it was back to feeling content without a new ambition as time passes us by. As Hemingway said, it is the journey that matters in the end, and having something new and exciting to strive for and work toward every day adds tremendous value to life, and contributes magnificently to the end result of attaining goals and making forward progress. It seems the issue is that we're setting goals that are too high and unreachable and we get discouraged when we don't achieve them, *and* that we're setting goals too low and we feel unfulfilled even when we attain them. So there's a sweet spot there, an untapped level of success, which we're missing because we haven't quite found the precise level of goal to aim for. Many people who have the initiative to set goals tend to look to role models who have achieved high levels of success and want to emulate them, following in their footsteps. This can be a source of inspiration but it can also be troublesome, deemed for failure.

I'm not trying to burst any bubbles or rain on anyone's parade, but you have to be real about who you are and how hard you're willing to work to achieve something that is only attained by a small percentage of people. Setting *achievable* goals, then, seems like the most reasonable action to take. How do we know what is achievable vs. unachievable? One way to look at it is to establish an outcome to attain, rather than try to emulate someone else's success. Are you more likely to get into really good shape—perhaps the best shape of your life, or be the next Mr. or Ms. Olympia (the title for the world's greatest bodybuilder)?

When we focus on emulating successful individuals, the level at which we have to perform is so high, it is all but impossible to achieve. The moment we focus on being *our* best, and reaching *our* potential, and capitalizing on *our* unique strengths, is when we really get somewhere with goal setting and achievement. The more we know about what we really want to achieve and *why* we want to achieve it, we can match that up with goals that are precisely within our range of attainment. Not too high, or too low, we can aim for them, work very hard, with a specific plan and even a timeline, and achieve meaningful outcomes. You have to believe in yourself and you have to be willing to work hard. No high level of success comes easy, even if it seems like it does in sports, on TV, or in movies. There is a lot of behind the scenes hard work that created every "overnight success." Taking the time to deliberately work through points A, B, C, and D en route to E, could make all the difference in your pursuit of meaningful goals.

You're not really that busy or that lazy. I want you to achieve your goals, and I am putting a special emphasis on that very desire. That's really what this is all about, empowering others to follow their passions and make *it* happen. Health and fitness goals can be attained if we approach them the right way and follow necessary actions to achieving them, even if some of them appear to be somewhat "lofty." There can still be time for social networking and downtime. Many aspects of personal entertainment can fit into your overall daily schedule, as long as health and fitness fit in there too. If aspects of health and fitness do not make it into your daily schedule, do something about it. Incorporate healthy foods and regular exercise into your routine in fun ways as a result of being well-prepared and aware of what foods and physical activities you enjoy. Then make time for them daily.

I challenge you to be anything but average, and to make a positive difference in your life and in the lives of those you care about. Aim to be remarkable, and live in ways that will make a lasting impression on others, literally creating a story worth positively remarking about. Go in the direction of your dreams even if it is against the grain, if you're willing to take a stand and put in the work to give yourself a solid chance at success.

Now that we got the reality of goal attainment out of the way, let's move on to how to set goals in the first place. This is an important step that cannot be missed, as it will set the tone for the rest of the book.

If you have only lost a few pounds over the past year, you cannot expect to lose 50 pounds next month alone (although you theoretically could, it would probably not be healthy weight loss and is not a sustainable method). If you weigh 150 pounds and are looking to bulk up, don't expect to weigh 200 pounds in eight weeks. There are methods and processes to achieve these goals that require a sincere desire to change, an action plan, a consistent schedule, and often other components such as a support network to help see you through. These objectives can be attained but each one will take time, patience and a lot of hard work.

How to create an attainable goal

Answer the following questions to get started:

1. What goal do you want to achieve? Be as detailed as possible in your answer and find a deep meaning behind it.

2. Why does it matter to you? You can't just say something like, "to look better." You have to address the root cause underlying your desires to "look better." So, why does it *really* matter to you?

3. What timeline are you setting for your goal? How did you determine this timeline? How does your reasoning match up with reality, science, and your actual daily schedule?

4. What three actions will you take each day to get you closer to achieving your goal? Be specific and select actions that are truly related to helping you get closer to your dream.

5. How are you going to measure your accountability?

6. How will your life change as a result of attaining your goal?

This is an example of one of my previous fitness goals, addressing each of these questions I asked of you.

Back in 1999 I was transitioning from distance running to bodybuilding. I will share my story with you of how setting a clear goal and following action steps with consistency helped me achieve something that initially didn't look like it was "in the cards" for me. I chose to share the following example because it is more on the extreme side, rather than just a simple goal of losing or gaining a few pounds. Simple goals are far more attainable, but I think you'll agree the example I am about to share is far more entertaining and inspiring.

I was always a skinny kid; through childhood and adolescence. All my life I was on the small and thin side, even through high school where I was a five-sport athlete. Though I grew up on a farm, ate plenty of high protein foods like most kids, and exercised a lot, I was a small guy. I weighed 89 pounds in eighth grade and barely over 100 pounds in my first year of high school. I got knocked around a lot on the soccer field and on the basketball court, but I was fast, and I used that to my advantage. After a successful high school athletic career that was built on the back of my speed and endurance, I ran cross country in college for the Beavers of Oregon State University. After one season of running cross country, I decided to pursue my dream of getting bigger and stronger, figuring it would open up doors for meaningful opportunities in my personal and professional life. Enter weightlifting and my introduction to the sport of bodybuilding. After a few pitfalls and shortcomings during my first year of weightlifting, for reasons I am fully aware of today, and speak about in my lectures throughout North America, I went back to my goal-setting roots to see me through this transition. My initial shortcomings were basically a result of not having a clear goal and not following action steps to achieve desired progress and success. I tried for a year to bulk up and ended up only gaining one pound. Not very awesome. Once I addressed and pursued this new goal with the right approach, I would not be stopped. Follow me back as I describe this specific goal in detail, addressing each of the six questions posed above.

Question #1:

What goal do you want to achieve? Be as detailed as possible in your answer and find a deep meaning behind it.

Answer:

In the summer of 2000, at a bodyweight of 157 pounds, I want to build up to at least 180 pounds within a year (summer of 2001) to be taken seriously as a bodybuilder. My whole life I have wanted to be bigger and stronger and I am now committed to make this happen through a nutrition and training program that will support my goals. Cutting back on running and incorporating weightlifting regularly will help me through this transformation process. Achieving this goal will improve my self-esteem, my self-confidence, and prove to myself that I am as hard of a worker in weightlifting as I have been in endurance running and academics, two areas I have excelled in. This will also make a profound statement for my vegan lifestyle, something that is very important to me. I want to represent the vegan fitness lifestyle in a positive and effective way so that others might become inspired to do the same.

Question #2:

Why does it matter to you? You can't just say something like, "to look better." You have to address the root cause underlying your desires to "look better." So, why does it *really* matter to you?

Answer:

This goal matters to me deeply because I am tired of being the little guy, I am tired of getting picked on, and I am tired of being overlooked. I have always wanted to be a professional wrestler, ever since I was eight years old, and achieving this muscle-building goal will get me closer to this dream than I have ever been before. I want to achieve this so badly I can taste it. I was born to lead by example and to achieve high levels of success, as I have proven in my life up to this point. This achievement will further validate my vegan lifestyle. Animals will be saved because of the influence this achievement will have on others. Nothing is going to get in my way. I will earn this through my commitment and dedication day in and day out.

Question #3:

What timeline are you setting for your goal? How did you determine this timeline? How does your reasoning match up with reality, science, and your actual daily schedule?

Answer:

This is the summer of 2000 and I will achieve my goal of weighing more than 180 pounds by the summer of 2001. I am giving myself a full year to gain a minimum of 23.1 pounds. (You know I'm focused on that .1). I am eager to achieve results fast, but I also know that I need to be patient and allow time for results to set in. A full year should be sufficient, given my level of commitment to this goal. I know I failed to reach my muscle-building goals last year, but I know what I did wrong and I have learned from my experiences. The previous time I attempted to build muscle I was only in the gym two or three days a week and I did not document my training or nutrition programs to have an accurate record of caloric intake and expenditure. I didn't give myself a real chance to grow. This time I will train six days per week with much more emphasis on nutrition and exercise recovery because I am aware of their direct connection to muscle development. I believe that with a consistent training schedule, and an increase in caloric intake with weekly evaluations of my progress, that I will achieve my goal. I am currently a student at the Utah College of Massage Therapy, the number one massage therapy school in the country, and I am learning about anatomy and physiology, biochemistry, sports nutrition, sports psychology, and other subjects directly related to understanding precisely how to alter my physique using proven scientific methods. My scientific understanding of muscle development will assist my real life muscle development. Though I am spending hours in classes in school, I am studying 7-10 hours per day, using a stopwatch to monitor my actual studying time, being totally transparent and completely accountable. I am working out every morning before 6:00 AM to ensure no matter what else happens during the day, I will know that I have held up my end of the deal in the gym. Academics directly impact my athletic outcome in my case. The more I know, the more I'll grow!

Question #4:

What three actions will you take each day to get you closer to achieving your goal? Be specific and select actions that are truly related to helping you get closer to your dream.

Answer:

1) I will complete roughly 50-100 push-ups and 50-100 crunches every single day, without exception. This will help me stay consistent with exercise and committed to making healthy, intelligent decisions on a regular basis. If I am willing to drop and give you 50-100 push-ups every single day, I am willing to eat the number of calories necessary to help me build muscle, and I am willing to get to the gym six days a week to train with intensity. This level of activity doing push-ups and crunches daily will not require me to take additional rest days from training because I will spread them out in numerous sets throughout the day, but will be a constant reminder that exercise is a top priority for me every day of the week.

Author's note: In reality, I ended up doing approximately 50-100 push-ups and crunches for 839 consecutive days (2.3 years without missing a day—even performing them on the floor in the corner at the Sundance Film Festival in Park City, UT, just to get them in to keep the streak alive).

2) I will read textbooks and study anatomy flash cards to help me understand in greater detail how my body responds and adapts to exercise, and I will apply what I learn in the gym, in the kitchen, and in the classroom.

3) I will refrain from using the Internet, no matter how much I want to get on Instant Messenger and flirt with girls that I hung out with in high school. That can wait until after graduation and after I attain my fitness goal, because I am working toward something meaningful that demands my attention every day.

Question #5:

How are you going to measure your accountability?

Answer:

I am going to be public about my goals. I will tell my classmates, even some of my teachers, what I will achieve. I will tell my friends and family what I am working toward and I will be transparent with my progress through all the ups and downs. My friends and classmates will see my commitment to excellence when I perform push-ups and crunches during breaks throughout the school day, and as they'll watch my body change from one month to the next. I will take any additional opportunities to meet with faculty during lunch breaks, days off, before and after school, to learn more about how to achieve this muscle-building goal while maintaining my status of academic leader in the school. Additionally, I will follow the Bill Phillip's Body-For-LIFE program and exercise six days per week and eat six meals per day, focusing on consuming quality protein, carbohydrates, fats, and sufficient water intake with each meal. This approach is more comprehensive and quantitative than any exercise program I have followed before. I look forward to objectively assessing my own accountability throughout this process.

Question #6:

How will your life change as a result of attaining your goal?

Answer:

My life will be better because I will have proven that I can achieve what others thought was impossible. This is the era of the late 1990s and early 2000s. I don't even know of any other vegan athletes, besides my classmate, Natalie, a yoga enthusiast who enjoys hiking.

My life will improve because I will have achieved a childhood dream of gaining lots of muscle (20+ pounds in a year), something I have never been able to successfully do. I will proudly share my vegan fitness lifestyle with those I encounter in school and in work. I will compete in a bodybuilding competition someday to be considered a "real" bodybuilder. I am committed to making this dream of building muscle as a vegan a reality, because, quite frankly, it just means a whole lot to me and I will do what it takes to make it happen. Challenge me. I will rise up to meet the challenge. Bring it on!

Conclusion and Results

You can see how I answered the questions that I presented to you. I hope my examples were clear and helpful. By now you're probably wondering how it all turned out. Well, here's what happened. My goal was grow from 157 pounds to over 180 pounds within a year, by the summer of 2001. In actuality, by the spring (April to be exact) of 2001 I weighed 185 pounds and started to cut fat to compete in my first bodybuilding competition a couple of months later with the goal of competing in the middle-weight division weighing under 176 pounds.

My goal was to gain 23.1 pounds in a year and I actually gained 28 pounds in ten months or so, before intentionally dropping weight to get shredded. A new goal to compete in bodybuilding superseded my bulking up goal, which I had already attained, so I changed directions based on my new passion, which dictated the direction I would go. I have no doubt that I achieved my goal *because* I addressed the six questions listed above. It is precisely because I created those action plans and answered meaningful questions that I was able to attain this muscle-building objective. Consistency, accountability and transparency were the catalysts that enabled me to achieve meaningful goals. This was more than a decade ago and I have followed this same system to achieve many positive outcomes in health, fitness, body-building, business, and in other areas of life. I simply chose to do what many people are often not willing to do, set attainable goals and work incredibly hard to achieve them.

Of course, it is easy for me to connect the dots after I already achieved the goal described above highlighting all the things I did right in order to succeed. The reality is, I knew what I needed to do in order to get to the end result I was seeking, and I followed these action steps because I knew the dots would connect in the future. I was aware that one outcome was depend-ent on a specific set of actions, and to reach my next result, new specific actions needed to be taken. This compounding formula is an effective way of ensuring your dots will connect in the future too. Visualize the future and think in terms of many steps ahead of where you are now to realize how each action has not only an immediate impact, but a residual impact that contributes progressively toward your destination. This approach can be taken with any new project, any new objective and any new goal. You can become aware of the dots that need to be connected ahead of time, and direct your actions to connect them, step-by-step, en route to achievement. I am creating new dots right now with this book, making connections with influential people while still in the writing process, and touring to key destinations, all with the objective to create dots that will connect once this book is released. What dots are you creating to connect in the future?

My vision is for you to learn, understand, and apply fundamental principles to achieving success. Now that you know what it means to be committed and to be transparent, burning fat, building muscle, and becoming a shredded plant-based athlete becomes simply a formula that you can follow if you can find it within yourself to say, "This matters to me, this is why, and this is what I'm going to do." I want you to succeed in whatever it is that moves you, whatever it is that you're passionate about, and whatever it is that you will pursue with all the enthusiasm you can muster. You must first believe in yourself and really mean it. From there, you're ahead of the game and poised for success.

Revisit the fundamental questions to ask yourself about why your goals matter at the beginning of this chapter, as well as the six questions requiring actions. When you find meaning in your pursuit, you will patiently go through points A, B, C, and D, and will arrive at your destination at point E having learned a lot along the way. Above all else, enjoy the ride.

– CHAPTER 3 –

Nutrition Basics –
An Introduction to Plant-Based Nutrition

> *"About eighty percent of the food on shelves*
> *of supermarkets today didn't exist 100 years ago."*
> — Larry McCleary

A general understanding of nutrition basics is helpful and makes the rest of the book easier to digest. This chapter will lay the groundwork for some common themes in health, wellness, and nutrition, such as the lists of macro and micronutrients and some insight into the roles they play in our overall health. Many people know that we should eat a lot of fruits and vegetables, but might not understand *why* we should eat them. This chapter aims to provide some insight into why these common health practices such as eating a variety of fruits, leafy green vegetables, and drinking sufficient quantities of water are relevant to our own personal health outcomes. Are carbohydrates to be avoided? How much protein do we really need? How do we know if we're eating enough or eating the right kinds of foods? We'll discuss these answers and more in this chapter and in greater depth in the next two chapters with regard to how these approaches impact the specific goals of burning fat and building muscle.

I studied nutrition in college, graduated from the Plant-Based Nutrition Certification Course through Cornell University, and have attended countless lectures by some of the leading doctors and nutritionists in the world. I have also watched hours upon hours of lectures online as well as professional DVDs, covering content related to health, wellness, nutrition, and exercise in an effort to enhance my own continued education. I recommend taking courses in this field as well to learn how your nutrition program can directly support your fitness goals in effective ways. I also suggest searching through the amazing free content online in the form of lectures and even accessible course material on the Internet. Make it a point to attend lectures in your community, travel to festivals and events such as the Holistic Holiday at Sea (vegan-friendly cruise), which highlights dozens of world-renowned health experts while also offering continuing education credits, and enroll in the now numerous online courses you can take to get a certification in plant-based nutrition, or similar credentials. You can find plant-based nutrition courses through the T. Colin Campbell Foundation, the McDougall Institute, The Wellness Forum and others. Many are listed in the resources in the back of the book. You will not only learn a lot, including life-saving information to share with your friends, family, colleagues, clients, and neighbors, but, like me, it can enhance your career and give you a more credible background in your areas of discourse. There are also weekend retreats, immersions, and intensive programs through The Engine 2 community, True North, and numerous other health and wellness communities specializing in the plant-based lifestyle. Take it as far as you want to, get as many certifications as you like, enroll in as many courses as you want, and above all else, put what you learn into action. Putting what you learn into action, and incorporating sound health practices in your day-to-day life, is a crucial step that is missed by many, including some experts. Why bother spending the time, energy, and often, money, to learn about lifesaving, health improving, performance-enhancing information if you're not going to use it?

We all know of experts in various fields who don't practice what they preach. Are they really any better off than the layperson that doesn't know quite as much but applies what they know in more productive ways? What if a heart surgeon knows all too well the risks involved in eating cholesterol-rich animal-based foods and the implications that has on plaque build-up in arteries and impending heart disease, but eats animal-based foods daily anyway? If the layperson understands the same health risks on a very basic level, and intentionally avoids consuming the artery-clogging foods as a result, and has lower cholesterol, less arterial wall blockage, and lower risk of heart disease, who is applying their knowledge more effectively? I give scenarios like this, and there are countless others I could list to parallel this notion, to show that just because someone is an expert doesn't always mean they lead by the best example. I believe the example itself is to be evaluated, not necessarily the background of the individual setting the example.

Just because someone is a nutritionist or registered dietitian, doesn't mean they necessarily follow the best health guidelines, or prescribe the best health guidelines to their patients and clients. Perhaps they have a blanket approach to all clients, suggesting eating an animal-based diet that likely causes disease, but advocate prescription drugs to offset the consumption of disease-causing foods. Would this be sound advice? Though I make it a point to evaluate the actions of experts, not just their words, at the same time, I am in no way suggesting you follow the advice of someone with no nutritional education or background, solely based on their physical or health appearance. There are plenty of factors at play that can lead to a desirable physical appearance, and a fit-looking exterior body doesn't always equate to a healthy interior body. What I am saying is that the application of effective health principles by individuals leading by a true positive example of health should not be overlooked. It is always a good idea to eat health-promoting plant-based whole foods. Putting a sound idea into action is the difference between understanding good health practices and applying good health practices. One does not need to be an expert to have superior health than an expert, based on nutrition and lifestyle practices alone. The fundamental basics of nutrition, such as the roles that macro and micronutrients play in our health, will always be the same, whether or not we follow sound nutrition principles. The nutritional science will be the same whether or not we adhere to it, and the better we understand the core nutritional concepts, the more intelligent health decisions we're likely to make.

If you currently follow a plant-based diet, you are no stranger to the "where do you get your protein?" question. Wouldn't it be nice to not only be able to identify plant-based whole-food protein sources, but perhaps ask the questioner if they can tell you the roles that protein plays in our health, and invite them to explain why protein is an important nutrient? When asked a question like this, many people will be stumped. Very likely, most of our friends, family members, and neighbors believe protein is not just important, but *especially* important, as if it is a magical potion, but they don't necessarily know *why* it is so important. A common guess is often, "because it helps the body stay strong," which is a pretty good answer, but it doesn't always reflect an accurate understanding of how the consumption of protein achieves that outcome. Having some basic knowledge of nutrition fundamentals will not only help you answer questions from your relatives at family gatherings during the holidays, but will give you a better understanding of how the food you eat directly relates to your health and athletic performance.

To understand the role that proper nutrition plays in our everyday lives, our athletic endeavors, and our long-term health, it is important to understand some basics. Having knowledge of some of the fundamental aspects of nutrition such as what protein, carbohydrates, fats, vitamins and minerals do will give us a better understanding of the importance of eating a clean, healthy diet.

Macronutrients

All food is made up of macronutrients and micronutrients. Macronutrients make up the bulk of the food we eat, somewhere between 95-99 percent of all food consumed. Macronutrients are commonly talked about among not just athletes, but many individuals. You may have heard friends say they are following an 80/10/10 diet for example. This is referring to the percentage of different macronutrients consumed per day. In this example, a minimum of 80 percent of calories come from carbohydrates, and a maximum of 10 percent each from proteins and fats. In the athletic world it is very common to discuss macronutrient percentages and athletes from dramatically different sports often have slightly different intake goals, based on how they believe their bodies will respond to the varied intake levels. A general rule to follow is to ensure the majority of your caloric intake comes in the form of carbohydrate-rich whole foods. Seventy to eighty percent of calories consumed each day should come from carbohydrates and 10-15 percent of calories coming from each proteins and fats. This is a standard approach to achieve high levels of health and wellness for athletes and non-athletes alike. For better or for worse, athletes tend to tweak these percentages based on their sport-specific goal. Strength athletes often significantly increase their percentage of calories from protein, endurance athletes commonly rely heavily on high levels of carbohydrates, and numerous types of athletes from varied sports backgrounds consume elevated levels of fats. I will argue over the next few chapters that it should not necessarily be the percentage of macronutrients that should be altered, but the volume of food within those same 80/10/10 or 70/15/15 percentages that should be changed based on the size and gender of the individual, their activity level, and caloric expenditure in relation to athletic goals.

Macronutrients are made up of:

Protein
Carbohydrates
Fats
Fiber*
Water*

These are the components that make up essentially all of our calories, and the percentages of the macronutrients we eat, is important. Sometimes alcohol is also on a macronutrient list because it contains calories, but it is nonessential, therefore it is often differentiated from the primary sources of calories. *Water is also required, but contains zero calories, therefore left off of many lists of macronutrients. It is a necessary substance for consumption, of course, and plays a major role in our overall health. *The same goes for fiber. It is a required nutrition component, but it is found in abundance in carbohydrate-rich foods and often not included with the "big three" on most lists. Therefore, you will likely see macronutrients listed on labels or charts comprised of just protein, carbohydrates, and fats. Each component has its benefits *and* consequences in times of over or under consumption. A diet that is made up of primarily whole food carbohydrates produces lots of energy. A diet comprised of mostly protein produces little energy and can lead to various kidney and liver problems, weight gain, and a host of other diseases. A diet made up of mostly fat will likely make the individual fat as well. Dr. John McDougall famously said, "The fat you eat is the fat you wear." Having a balance is important, but the right balance is what is most important. Not just one third of each major macronutrient, but understanding the appropriate percentages for consumption based on necessity and health outcome. An approach I take is approximately 70/15/15, referring to 70 percent of daily calories from (whole food) carbohydrates and 15 percent each from proteins and fats. These numbers are well within healthy ranges and are about as close to ideal for energy production, muscle recovery and growth, joint care, digestion and assimilation ease, and disease prevention as you can get. Anywhere within a few percentage points of these numbers, while avoiding alcohol, which is just empty calories leading to fat gain, and potentially other associated problems, is an effective approach to take.

The reason I prefer this specific ratio is because I believe that if your whole-food, plant-based diet truly is diverse, your diet will consist of a combination of many high carbohydrate foods such as fruits, vegetables and grains, some high protein foods such as legumes, nuts and green leafy vegetables, and some high fat foods such as nuts and seeds and certain fruits like avocados. With a truly diverse diet that includes a broad spectrum of food groups, an 80/10/10 outcome is harder to attain and not as practical. Likewise, a carbohydrate intake under 70 percent is less likely when consuming only whole foods, avoiding concentrated nutrients from high levels of proteins and fats found in many processed foods. Therefore, a 70/15/15 target seems to be the most natural, most practical, convenient and healthy approach that I know of, and it makes sense to implement a guideline that is close to these macronutrient targets.

You can see from the list below how many calories are associated with a single gram of each of the macronutrients. Based on these numbers alone, you can see why we run into health problems when our fat intake is up around 35 percent of our total calories, which is the American average. It is no wonder that statistically, most people in America (and in nations with similar fat intake) are overweight and have health problems as a result. These negative health implications can be avoided and even reversed when a new approach takes its place, such as 15 percent fat intake rather than 35 percent or more, which is the current "standard" for many.

> Protein = 4 calories per gram
> Carbohydrates = 4 calories per gram
> Alcohol = 7 calories per gram
> Fats = 9 calories per gram

Upon digestion, absorption, and metabolism, macronutrients yield energy (carbohydrates and fats) and provide specialized biological functions. They are absorbed in the intestines and then go into the bloodstream. There they are transported, most often to the liver, to be used and metabolized. Carbohydrates are our primary fuel source, followed by fats and then proteins.

To help give you fuel (pun intended) for your debates with your relatives about proper nutrition, the following are some of the important roles that macronutrients play. These lists were provided by the McKinley Health Center at the University of Illinois at Urbana-Champaign:

Source: http://www.mckinley.illinois.edu/handouts/macronutrients.htm

Protein

- Growth (especially important for children, teens, and pregnant women)
- Tissue repair
- Immune function
- Making essential hormones and enzymes
- Energy when carbohydrate is not available
- Preserving lean muscle mass

Carbohydrates

- The body's main source of fuel

- Easily used by the body for energy

- All of the tissues and cells in our body can use glucose for energy

- Needed for the central nervous system, the kidneys, the brain, the muscles (including the heart) to function properly

- Can be stored in the muscles and liver and later used for energy

- Important in intestinal health and waste elimination

Fat

- Normal growth and development

- Energy (fat is the most concentrated source of energy)

- Absorbing certain vitamins (like vitamins A, D, E, K, and carotenoids)

- Providing cushioning for the organs

- Maintaining cell membranes

- Providing taste, consistency, and stability to foods

Now you know the roles that these macronutrients play in our everyday health so you can have a better understanding of why they are important as you construct your own personal nutrition program. When you understand the role that protein plays in your health you will know that more isn't necessarily better, in fact, more protein is often worse for our health. With this proper nutritional understanding we can see how silly the obsession with high protein really is. It is not only a rather obnoxious and unwarranted focal point in nutrition, it is a dangerous one with myriad adverse side effects when too much is consumed.

Source: http://nutritionfacts.org/video/do-vegetarians-get-enough-protein/

Micronutrients

Micronutrients are vitamins and minerals. They make up just a small percentage of the food we take in but play a crucial role in keeping our bodies healthy. They are absolutely necessary to sustain life. Whole plant foods are filled with micronutrients but there should not be an emphasis on consuming singular nutrients (eating foods specifically high in Vitamin C or Vitamin K or any other particular vitamin) or isolated nutrients, extracted and added to other foods. Simply, a balanced diet of fruits, vegetables, nuts, grains, seeds and legumes will provide sufficient micronutrient diversity and quantities, assuming one has adequate caloric intake. Aside from specific medical conditions, there is no need to consume 1,000 percent of your Recommended Daily Allowance of a specific micronutrient. You wouldn't easily find numbers of that scale in nature and there is rarely ever a need for such an extreme level of consumption. Yet, thousands of products have isolated nutrients injected into foods to reveal hundreds of percentage points, or even thousands of percentage points of the RDA of a vitamin or mineral in their product. At a mainstream grocery store I recently saw a product advertising 10,000% RDA of a specific vitamin. Are you kidding me? There is no natural reason to ingest vitamin or mineral contents of that level and you likely won't find a plant in nature that produces such an extreme intake level in a single serving. There are numerous health risks with consuming too high or too low levels of specific nutrients, and getting natural intake levels from a diversity of real foods, should be practical and sufficient. You can always get blood work done to check your own micronutrient levels and if numbers are high or low in a given area you can adjust your nutrition intake accordingly. Eat more walnuts or flax seeds if Omega-3 essential fatty acids are low. Consume more nuts and legumes if your levels of zinc are low, and so on. You shouldn't have to go too far out of your way, as a diverse whole-food diet comprised of your favorite foods will be nutritionally adequate, and will also be nutritionally superior to common processed food and animal-based diets.

Though it is not important to isolate individual nutrients, a list of vitamins and minerals are listed below as a reference to understand what they are and what they do. If you do happen to have high or low levels of any of these micronutrients, based on blood test results, you can simply alter your diet by searching which foods contain various levels, and increase or decrease consumption of such foods based on that data. Once you have a general awareness of where certain nutrients come from in whole foods, make a concerted effort to include them, just as you would make an effort to include a diversity of adequate calories and sufficient water intake every day. The only time a focused effort has to be made to consume specific foods that contain specific levels of desired nutrients is when you know, based on real data, that you are significantly high or low in some areas. Just as we know we need to reduce cholesterol intake when we have high cholesterol levels, and take action to bring them down to healthy levels, the same could be said for boosting levels of Omega-3 consumption, increased sun exposure to raise levels of Vitamin D, or some other targeted behavior to achieve a desired health outcome. Aside from specific scenarios such as those outlined above, a true balanced whole-food, plant-based diet with diversity of foods from all major plant-food categories should not only be sufficient, it should be a more desirable and complete nutrition plan than you've ever followed before. Never underestimate the value of diversity and variety coming from nature's original foods—plants.

Vitamins are organic substances made by carbon, usually produced by plants. There are water soluble and fat soluble vitamins. Minerals are inorganic compounds needed by plants and animals for proper growth and functioning.

Water Soluble   **Fat Soluble**

Vitamin C   Vitamins A, D, E, K
B Vitamins

Minerals

Calcium	Bone structure
Iron	Blood function (hemoglobin)
Zinc	Aid in controlling enzyme reactions
Magnesium	Bone structure
Selenium	Aid in controlling enzyme reactions
Sodium	Maintain fluid balance
Potassium	Maintain fluid balance

Vitamin B12

Vitamins are found in abundance in plant-based whole foods, except for one very important one, which is an organic compound that is attained in the diet through the consumption of bacteria. This vitamin is Vitamin B12. Vitamin B12 is a required nutrient necessary for brain function and many other important roles in our overall health. It is often found in bacteria present in red meat, therefore people who avoid red meat and animal products in general, tend to either have low levels of Vitamin B12 and/or are required to supplement with cyanocobolamin or methylcobalamin (the two common forms of Vitamin B12). Vitamin B12 supplementation is advised for everyone who is not eating animal products covered in bacteria. We live in a society where our food and water supply are very sterile and we are unlikely to get sufficient levels of Vitamin B12 from the bacteria around us.

Supplementation is highly advised. The consensus among the top doctors and nutritionists referenced throughout this book (Dr. T. Colin Campbell, Dr. Michael Greger, Dr. Matthew Lederman, Dr. Alona Pulde, and many others) is that everyone following a plant-based diet should supplement with Vitamin B12. When it comes to something so important (having an impact on brain and nerve function), I always advise siding with the world renowned experts, which is in your best health interest. Though many vegan foods are fortified with Vitamin B12, I advocate a whole food approach, which does not often include such processed, fortified foods, including non-dairy milks, breads, cereals, and canned and packaged foods. Therefore, when plant-based whole foods are truly at the foundation of one's diet, making up the bulk of calories consumed on a daily basis, Vitamin B12 supplementation is all but required and highly recommended.

According to the Harvard Medical School for Harvard Health Publications, "The human body needs vitamin B_{12} to make red blood cells, nerves, DNA, and carry out other functions. The average adult should get 2.4 micrograms a day. Like most vitamins, B_{12} can't be made by the body. Instead, it must be gotten from food or supplements. And therein lies the problem: Some people don't consume enough vitamin B_{12} to meet their needs, while others can't absorb enough, no matter how much they take in. As a result, vitamin B_{12} deficiency is relatively common, especially among older people. The National Health and Nutrition Examination Survey estimated that 3.2 percent of adults over age 50 have a seriously low B_{12} level, and up to 20 percent may have a borderline deficiency."

Source: http://www.health.harvard.edu/blog/
vitamin-b12-deficiency- can-be-sneaky-harmful-201301105780

According to internationally recognized physician and bestselling author, Dr. Michael Greger, from the acclaimed medical website, www.nutritionfacts. org, people should supplement with Vitamin B12 daily or weekly with specific amounts. His thoughts include, "In my professional opinion, the easiest and most inexpensive way to get one's B-12 is to take at least 2,500mcg (μg) of cyanocobalamin once each week, ideally as a chewable, sublingual, or liquid supplement (you can't take too much–all you get is expensive pee).

"Or, if you'd rather get into the habit of taking something daily (instead of once-a-week), I recommend at least 250mcg (I know the math doesn't 'add up' but that's due to the vagaries of the B-12 receptor system.)

"Or, if you'd rather get it from B-12-fortified foods instead of supplements, I'd suggest three servings a day, each containing at least 25% of the 'Daily Value' on its label."

Source: http://nutritionfacts.org/2011/08/30/3964/

Whether you supplement with cyanocobalamin or methylcobalamin, the important thing is to take some sort of a Vitamin B12 supplement on a daily or weekly basis to be proactive and avoid potential risks of sustaining low levels and the consequences associated with such an outcome. I start my morning with 500mg of methylcobalamin every day through a supplemental Vitamin B12 spray under my tongue, because I believe it absorbs more efficiently when taken sublingually. I prefer methylcobalamin because I understand it to have higher and easier absorption rates than cyanocobalamin, though either should get the job done as long as you consume it regularly. I realize that is somewhat on the high end of consumption, but nerve, joint, and cognitive issues are not something I am willing to jeopardize or mess around with. You shouldn't either. Supplement with Vitamin B12 and take it seriously and encourage your plant-based and vegan friends to do the same, especially if they are following a whole-food diet, not relying on processed foods, which may or may not be sufficiently fortified. Vitamin B12 is the only supplement I have used consistently over the past two years; essentially all of my other nutrition comes from plant-based whole foods.

Vitamin D

If you live in latitude areas above Los Angeles, Dallas, Atlanta and others cities throughout the world that correspond with those latitudinal planes, you may run the risk of having low levels of Vitamin D. We manufacture Vitamin D primarily through our exposure to the sun, and if you live in an area of the world that doesn't get very much sun for months on end, such as most U.S. states, all of Canada, most of Europe, and parts of Asia, during the winter months, it would behoove you to either take a vacation somewhere sunny or take a Vitamin D supplement.

The Harvard School of Public Health has this to say about Vitamin D:

"If you live north of the line connecting San Francisco to Philadelphia and Athens to Beijing, odds are that you don't get enough vitamin D. The same holds true if you don't get outside for at least a 15-minute daily walk in the sun. African-Americans and others with dark skin, as well as older individuals, tend to have much lower levels of vitamin D, as do people who are overweight or obese.

"Worldwide, an estimated 1 billion people have inadequate levels of vitamin D in their blood, and deficiencies can be found in all ethnicities and age groups. Indeed, in industrialized countries, doctors are even seeing the resurgence of rickets, the bone-weakening disease that had been largely eradicated through vitamin D fortification.

"Why are these widespread vitamin D deficiencies of such great concern? Because research conducted over the past decade suggests that vitamin D plays a much broader disease-fighting role than once thought.

"Being 'D-ficient' may increase the risk of a host of chronic diseases, such as osteoporosis, heart disease, some cancers, and multiple sclerosis, as well as infectious diseases, such as tuberculosis and even the seasonal flu.

"Currently, there's scientific debate about how much vitamin D people need each day. The Institute of Medicine, in a long-awaited report released on November 30, 2010 recommends tripling the daily vitamin D intake for children and adults in the U.S. and Canada, to 600 IU per day. The report also recognized the safety of vitamin D by increasing the upper limit from 2,000 to 4,000 IU per day, and acknowledged that even at 4,000 IU per day, there was no good evidence of harm. The new guidelines, however, are overly conservative about the recommended intake, and they do not give enough weight to some of the latest science on vitamin D and health. For bone health and chronic disease prevention, many people are likely to need more vitamin D than even these new government guidelines recommend."

Source: http://www.hsph.harvard.edu/nutritionsource/vitamin-d/

Like Vitamin B12, Vitamin D consumption should not be overlooked, especially if you live in places with long winters. If you have low levels of Vitamin D, start a coin jar and save for a sunny vacation or simply supplement with the figures that Harvard suggests or what Dr. Michael Greger suggests on www.nutritionfacts.org.

I don't take Vitamin D supplements because I live a nomadic lifestyle and have favorite sunny destinations I frequent yearly including California, Arizona, Nevada, Texas, Florida, Mexico, and the Caribbean loading up on my calcium absorbing-enhancing Vitamin D. I currently live in Colorado, known for its 300 days of sun per year, and when weather permits, I prefer to exercise outdoors. Let this be your motivation to get out there and explore. Soak up the sun in the name of good health.

Metabolism

Metabolism is the act of transforming absorbed nutrients into products that fulfill specialized functions such as producing enzymes, and producing factors that are used in immune function. It occurs after digestion and absorption and is known for many functions, especially for producing energy and acting as antioxidants. Metabolism is also your body's mechanism for burning fat (a method of producing energy). Some people have a faster metabolism than others and whether fast or slow, both have pros and cons. Your rate of metabolism will change based on numerous factors such as your age, gender, and lifestyle. If you increase or decrease your meal frequency or alter your activity level, you will likely have a measurable impact on your rate of metabolism. If you eat low nutrient-dense foods or high nutrient-dense foods, that reality can have an impact on your metabolism. Even the amount of water you consume each day could have an influence on your rate of metabolism.

Being able to control metabolism to some degree, and observe these changes can be helpful and inspiring. This is what can get an athlete really excited about how the body utilizes what we give it to help us perform. Learning how to produce and conserve energy is an important lesson in creating an efficient system to achieve high levels of athletic success. Consuming smaller meals and eating more frequently can speed up metabolism, as can being more physically active in general and drinking lots of water, say a gallon a day. Likewise, few meals spread out throughout the day and inactivity can slow metabolism. A faster metabolism will lead to burning fat at a more efficient rate, likely fighting off numerous diseases such as obesity and side effects that come with that disease, but a slower metabolism has been linked to greater longevity. In essence, it seems to slow down our aging process to a degree. Surely, we experience a flux of faster and slower rates of metabolism throughout our lifetime, and you can look into what specific approaches fulfill your personal health interests. A balanced diet of whole plant food meals throughout the day combined with an active lifestyle is always a healthy recommendation for anyone.

Additional Notes

There are plenty of other aspects of nutrition we could cover from antioxidants to fiber, to ATP Transport, cell nutrition, immune system support, and the list goes on. This has been a basic overview of some of the fundamental principles in nutrition that are most commonly on the minds of athletes (calories, protein, carbohydrates, amino acids, vitamins, recovery, and performance). For more in depth information regarding any aspect of nutrition, refer to more specialized books on those subject matters. A few recommendations include *Becoming Vegan* by Registered Dietitians Brenda Davis and Vesanto Melina, *The China Study* by Dr. T. Colin Campbell, *Eat To Live* by Dr. Joel Fuhrman, and *Basic Course in Vegetarian and Vegan Nutrition* by George Eisman, RD. Really, any book on nutrition will give you a good understanding of general concepts like energy production, metabolism, the role of macronutrients, micronutrients, antioxidants, and similar topics. In the plant-based community, there are many world-renowned health and medical specialists including Dr. John McDougall, Dr. Caldwell Esselstyn, Dr. Matthew Lederman, Dr. Alona Pulde, Dr. Pam Popper, Dr. Neal Barnard, Dr. Michael Greger, Dr. Michael Klaper, and numerous others you can look into for more detailed information. There are some outstanding plant-based Registered Dietitians as well, including George Eisman, Jeff Novick, Julieanna Hever, Jack Norris, Matt Ruscigno, and Ginny Messina who have popular books and helpful websites. An entire directory of doctors, dietitians, trainers, and experts is listed in the back of this book.

My goal with this chapter is to get you some basic nutritional information for you to apply in your own fat-burning and muscle-building programs. I know from experience that when I learned some basics, *and* applied what I learned, I progressed at a much faster rate than I did previously without a basic understanding of human nutrition. Many of my colleagues have experienced the same outcome through increased knowledge in this discipline.

Nutrition Basics Summary

As stated earlier, although it is good to know the roles that individual nutrients play, you need not focus on individual nutrient consumption unless you have a clinical deficiency that needs to be corrected. There should not be an emphasis on foods high in protein, high in carbohydrates, high in fats, or high in a specific vitamin or mineral, but an emphasis on eating a diversity of whole foods, which naturally contain a balanced and healthy amount of all of these nutrients in a sufficient, varied, and healthy diet. Though we aim to attain macronutrient consumption of roughly 70/15/15 for good overall health and athletic performance, all we have to do to achieve this is to eat produce and avoid processed, isolated, and concentrated foods. Whole plant foods naturally have high levels of carbohydrates and are generally low in fat and protein. The human body is so complex and so sophisticated that it can apply what you give it to perform incredible functions to keep you healthy, strong, and thriving in your active lifestyle. Eat your favorite plant-based whole foods with some effort focused on diversity so you're not eating the same few foods every day, and you will be well on your way to fueling a machine ready to perform at a high level in whatever fitness discipline you pursue.

Remember, true health isn't about what we *think* we're eating or how we *think* we're exercising and the healthy habits we *believe* we have, but it is the result of our *true* actions. That is why consistency, accountability, and transparency are so incredibly important. Don't just talk about exercising regularly and eating healthy foods. Do it.

Also, remember to drink lots of water, especially if you're active. Seventy percent of our bodies are comprised of water. Don't just talk about drinking sufficient quantities. Do it. This is especially important if you are very active, exercise regularly, or live in a warm climate. Stay nourished and hydrated to be at your best. A gallon a day might seem like a lot of water to consume, but it could also be a single action that helps improve numerous health situations. From better cell nutrition to nourished organs, to flushing out toxins from the body, to reducing the risk of cramping during or after exercise; consuming a gallon of water a day should be a goal for all of us. Your brain is also made of up seventy percent water so if you have an academic challenge ahead of you, or simply want to support your cognitive functions the best you can, cheers, drink up.

Discover your own particular interests in nutrition and take courses, study, and attend lectures to learn more. Learn from those who truly lead by example, from what they say to how they live. Most importantly, apply what you learn and lead by a positive example so that others may learn from your experiences too. Don't eat to get by, eat to thrive.

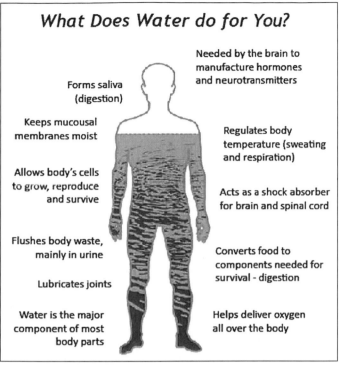

You are made up of 70% water. Drink up!
Courtesy of water.usgs.gov

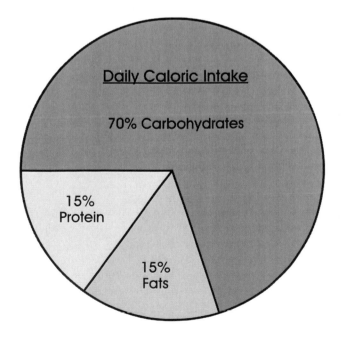

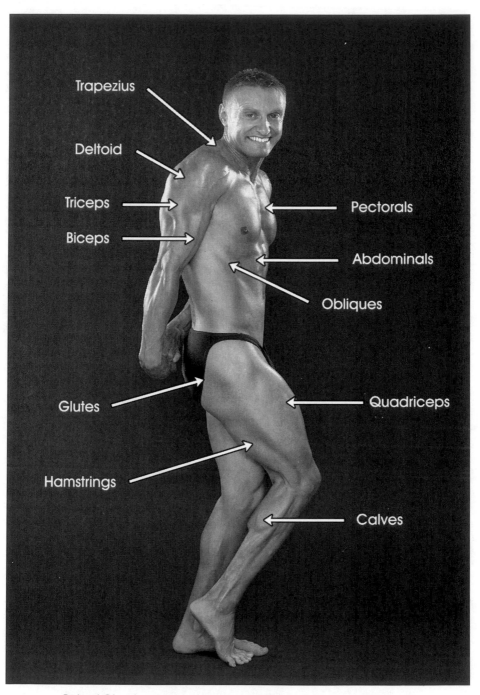

Robert Cheeke - Photo by Melissa Schwartz - theveganrevolution.net

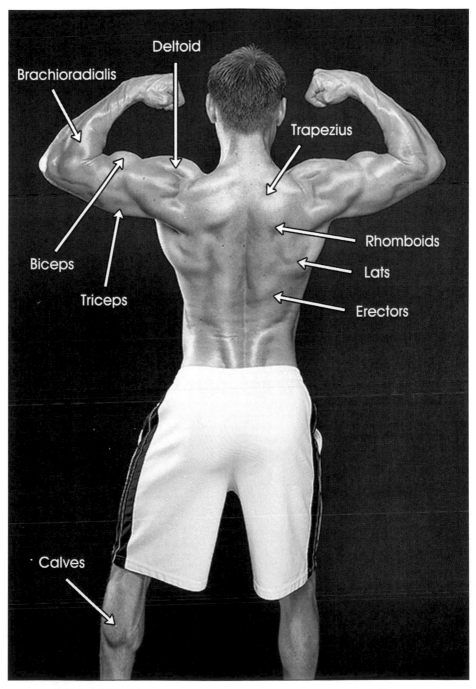

Robert Cheeke - Photo by Melissa Schwartz - theveganrevolution.net

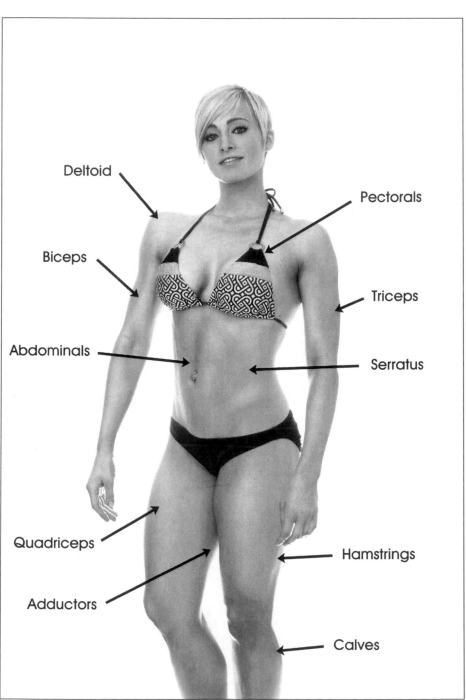

Deltoid

Pectorals

Biceps

Triceps

Abdominals

Serratus

Quadriceps

Hamstrings

Adductors

Calves

Mindy Collette

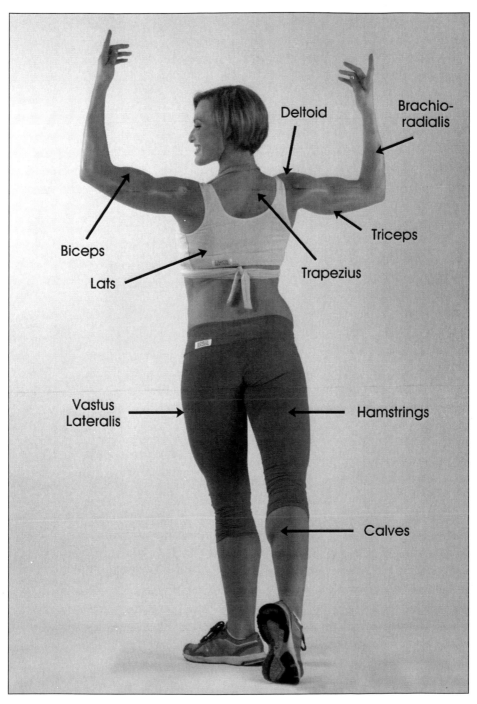

Deltoid

Brachio-
radialis

Biceps

Triceps

Lats

Trapezius

Vastus
Lateralis

Hamstrings

Calves

Mindy Collette

– CHAPTER 4 –

Burning Fat Efficiently

> *"If it doesn't challenge you, it won't change you."*
> — Fred Devito, yoga instructor

A
s I stated earlier, most people really do want to lose fat, they just don't know how to effectively do it. In this chapter I will break down precisely how you can alter your training and nutrition programs in ways that will effectively burn fat so you can achieve your weight-loss and fat-loss goals. There are three distinct fat-loss topics I will write about including:

1. Exercising first thing in the morning on an empty stomach to get into an optimal fat-burning zone. Multiple other training methods such as High Intensity Interval Training (HIIT) and aerobic exercise following weight training are additional quality methods to achieve fat-loss.

2. Why what we eat before, during, and after exercise could be one of the most telling factors as to whether or not we will be able to burn fat. The role of nutrition timing is an essential part of a fat-loss program because it can have a direct correlation to progression or regression in relation to goals.

3. Why understanding the difference between caloric density and nutrient density might be one of the greatest oversights by those who are trying to burn fat but are hitting plateaus. Identifying your own Basal Metabolic Rate (BMR) by using a Harris-Benedict calculator, discussed in detail in Chapter 5, could quite literally make the difference between success and failure in fat-loss and will open your eyes to solutions for problems you have run into in the past.

Fat-burning Training

You have seen people at the gym running on the treadmill for twenty or thirty minutes, riding a bike for half an hour, or simply going for a forty-five minute walk, all in the name of burning fat and losing weight. These individuals are hard to miss. They are often watching television, talking with a friend while they train, or perhaps even having a cell phone conversation while trying not to fall off the treadmill. Equipped with a neon-colored sports drink in hand, they are on a mission to burn fat to finally achieve their New Year's Resolutions and lose weight. Do you notice any problems with this picture? These individuals could very well be committed, performing these exercises five days per week and still not see fat-loss results. How can this be? With a consistent program performing aerobic exercise, it should be an ideal environment for fat-burning. The problem with this approach is that most people have it all wrong when it comes to understanding how the body burns fat. While all of those approaches *could* lead to fat burning under the right circumstances, they are rarely effective. The problem lies in a few key areas that make a big difference.

The treadmill runner usually eats food within an hour or two before their half-hour training session and has stored carbohydrates (from food consumption) to burn through before ever getting into a fat-burning zone, which uses fat as its fuel. Since carbohydrates are the primary fuel source, the body will burn carbohydrates for fuel rather than fat. The runner does not stay on the treadmill long enough to burn through stored carbohydrates (calories from foods and beverages consumed) to get to a situation in which the body then turns to fat as its fuel source. If the runner does not run long enough, or fast enough (accelerating the calorie-burning process), he or she will not get into an effective fat-burning zone. The runner may tone their legs and strengthen their heart and lungs with their effort, but will have missed the opportunity to burn fat, which is often their primary goal for the aerobic exercise in the first place. You can now see why running on a treadmill everyday can still be an ineffective method of burning fat when the environment for fat-burning is not present. The calories consumed beforehand often prevent fat-burning from taking place if the duration of exercise is too short of a period. Had the treadmill runner spent an hour or more on the treadmill from an extended conversation with their neighbor, or if they couldn't bear to get off the treadmill before their favorite TV show was over, or had run at an accelerated pace for the half hour (to burn more calories per minute), the situation could be quite different, as I will outline below.

The person on the stationary bike may or may not have eaten within a couple of hours before the workout, but could be sipping on a sugary drink, adding more carbohydrates to their system to have to burn through before calling upon stored fat as fuel. Drinking a calorically-dense sugary beverage for "energy" during cardiovascular training with the goal of burning fat is like eating cake for breakfast as part of your weight-loss program. It does not make any sense if fat burning is the goal. If just getting through the workout is the objective, and additional fuel is needed to combat fatigue, a natural energy drink or another fuel source such as fruit will do nicely. But this should be avoided regardless of the type of exercise you are doing if you are trying to burn fat.

The walker might not be burning enough total calories during their stroll to elicit a change from carbohydrates to fat as their primary fuel source during their walk. Let's be honest, most people don't just go for a walk without playing on their smart phone, making a phone call, or finding some other distraction to focus on other than the exercise task at hand. If they ate within an hour or so of their walk and/or eat or drink during their walk, which many people tend to do, they certainly will not be using fat as a primary fuel source. They will still be burning through recently consumed calories. This clearly does not support their fat loss efforts. They might have good intentions, but intentions don't lead to the achievement of goals, actions do.

In all of these scenarios we can clearly see where the individual went wrong in their pursuit of burning fat. Using these same scenarios, how can we change the circumstances to get the individual into a proper and effective fat-burning zone? The treadmill runner could avoid eating a couple of hours before exercising, or even better, run on an empty stomach first thing in the morning upon waking. Since they will not have carbohydrates readily available from recently consumed calories, their bodies will naturally call upon fat as fuel and burn fat during their workout. The cyclist can use the same approach to training on an empty stomach and avoid consuming sugary drinks or other calories during their workout. The walker could jog during parts of their exercise to accelerate calorie burning or could walk for a longer period to ensure they burn through stored carbohydrates to use fat as fuel. The walker could also walk up hill or up various flights of stairs to increase their caloric expenditure per minute. Or they could just stay off their phone so they can focus on pace, distance, and breathing efficiently to get closer to success. All of these scenarios (treadmill running, cycling, and walking) *can* work for fat burning, but they usually don't, for the reasons outlined above. There are some general principles to understand and apply in your own pursuit to burn fat, a goal that most of the population shares. The following are some helpful, and perhaps life-changing, tips to incorporate into your own exercise program, and to share with others who are struggling to attain their fat-loss goals.

Unless you surpass an hour of continuous exercise, or exercise on an empty stomach first thing in the morning, or do aerobic exercise at a very high intensity, you are still likely using carbohydrates as primary fuel, and not burning fat. You may tone your legs and strengthen your heart and lungs with your 20-45 minute exercise sessions, but you are not getting into an ideal fat-burning zone if the exercise length or level of intensity does not match your objective, or if you are eating or drinking calories during exercise. There is a very clear explanation for why those who exercise regularly, but for short durations, are unable to achieve their fat-loss goals. The frustration that comes from stagnant fat loss does not have to continue. This chapter will cover a variety of solutions to this health problem that impacts many of our friends, family members, and neighbors. First, though, we must understand how science works in our approach to our fitness goals, in this case, fat reduction and weight loss.

When we eat food, which is mostly made up of carbohydrates—aside from animal-based foods, which are primarily made up of protein and fat— we store carbohydrates in the form of glycogen to be used as fuel. When we exercise, we call upon these glycogen stores to provide us energy for exercise, or any physical activity, for that matter. After a meal is consumed, and a period of time for digestion between consumption and exercise passes, we begin our physical activity. When we initiate exercise, we have about an hour's worth of carbohydrate stores to fuel our continuous athletic activity. Clearly, some sports take much longer than an hour to play or engage in. Major team sports such as basketball, football, soccer, and baseball, as well as marathon running, immediately come to mind. It is within these sports and many others of similar duration that you will notice athletes consuming sugary drinks, snacks, fruit, and other energy-producing foods during exercise (during a time-out in basketball, halftime of a soccer match, and at marathon aid stations, for example). These refuel the body with carbohydrates, electrolytes, and other nutrients to keep going, just as we refuel with snacks and a lunch break at work to keep ourselves energized through the workday. This does not, however, help us burn fat. If we know we have about one hour of readily available carbohydrate fuel to use, what happens after we surpass an hour and do not take in any additional calories? Our bodies will turn to the second most efficient fuel source we have, which is fat, as fuel. Therefore, if we exercise for more than an hour (I prefer one hour and fifteen minutes to be sure I have burned through all available carbohydrates when fat-burning is my primary goal), and then continue exercising for an additional 15-30 minutes, that period is our fat-burning zone. Do you often see overweight marathon runners or heavy Tour de France cyclists? Probably not. That is because they are exercising for such a long time, they naturally get into a fat-burning zone regularly. They train for long periods on a consistent basis, for more than an hour before refueling, and their bodies adapt to this workload over time, shedding fat and building up a strong aerobic capacity. Anything beyond an additional hour (two total hours) without taking in calories can be counter-productive and unhealthy. You also run the risk of significant fatigue, dehydration, and cramping by going multiple hours without the consumption of anything but water, which has zero calories, or fuel. Cyclists and marathon runners often consume snacks during their exceptionally long training sessions, and use those calories as fuel they burn through, so they don't get stored as fat. Most of us probably overeat due to the increased appetite that exercise induces, but don't burn off those excess calories, therefore end up storing fat, even when we exercise fairly regularly.

A great approach is to engage in whatever sports interest you have for an hour or so, and then go for a jog for half an hour after that. If you don't know what type of fat-burning cardiovascular exercise to do, evaluate your own interests to determine what you really like to do. You will discover that some activities you didn't even associate with "exercise" do indeed burn a lot of calories (hiking, skiing, kayaking, dancing, and sand volleyball to name a few). Even if your answer is playing laser tag, you are being transparent, you've discovered what you really enjoy, and you'll get a high five from me, because laser tag totally rocks! If running is your primary sports interest, finish your workout and go for a cool down jog or walk afterwards. My personal favorite approach is to lift weights for about an hour to an hour and fifteen minutes, and then jog, hike, cycle or walk for 15-30 minutes after that. If I am living in a cold climate (rare, because I am obsessed with the sun and tropical locations), or if it is winter and my training will be mostly indoors, I use the stair-stepper or stationary bike for my fat-burning cardiovascular conditioning after weight training. If team sports are more your thing, playing an extra game of basketball or jogging around kicking a soccer ball for fun or simply playing catch with a football or baseball, running after a ball as a "cool down" after your primary workout, is a nice fat-burning, low-impact activity. Playing chess or poker doesn't count. Sorry, Daniel Negreanu (2013 World Series of Poker Player of The Year – and vegan), you're going to have to do something else besides take my money in a Texas hold 'em game to burn sufficient calories. A round of golf isn't much better, but is a step in the right direction.

Part of the objective is to make fat-burning exercise fun, so finding something that is truly enjoyable to you is a major key. If it is not fun, you will likely skip exercise all together, missing out on what may be the most beneficial action step in achieving your goals. List all your favorite physical activities, from swimming to throwing a Frisbee for your dog, and everything in between, and make it a point to make fun, fat-burning exercise a priority. When it comes to exercise, I promise you, if you don't enjoy it, you won't do it for a prolonged period (which is often what is necessary to see results), and if you truly love it, you will find ways to do it. So it is imperative that you find something that makes you smile. Are there any rock climbers out there? (A fun, physically-demanding activity. I suggest you try it.) Or if you take playing table tennis or air hockey as seriously as I do, you'll work up more of a sweat doing those activities than many people who are exercising in a gym will.

Note – Use this online calculator to learn how many calories you will burn during a given exercise. This can help you choose which exercises to engage in based on your fat-burning objectives compared with your true interests, or simply reveal the caloric expenditure of your current exercise routine based on your bodyweight and intensity level of the given exercise: http://www.healthstatus.com/calculate/cbc

What if you're like a lot of people and don't have an hour or two to spend exercising each day? What if 90 minutes out of your 1,440 minutes per day is too much to ask to spend improving your health and achieving your goals? Well, you are in luck. You can expedite the calorie-burning process by increasing the intensity of your exercise. You may have heard of High Intensity Training (HIT) or High Intensity Interval Training (HIIT) before. Basically what this means is that rather than standing, sitting, or otherwise resting between sets, you make exercise continuous. For example, if you would normally lift weights and then take a seat on a bench for a minute or two before completing your next set, when you are training with a HIT style, you would finish your lifting set and then immediately jump rope or perform some other high impact aerobic exercise to keep your heart rate up and accelerate calorie-burning. If your normal weightlifting workout would burn 400 calories in an hour, a HIT workout could exceed 800 calories burned during the same time period depending on level of intensity. That is double the calories burned, simply by altering your training style in a way that can be really fun too. If you haven't tried HIT, or other similar styles of training such as CrossFit, I highly recommend that you experience them soon. You can see how a HIT approach can burn through stored glycogen fuel quickly and get your body into a fat-burning zone much faster than a lower intensity workout.

When running for 15-30 minutes every day does not do anything for fat-burning if the circumstances are not right, try running (or any other preferred exercise) for 90 minutes a day, just a few days a week, and see what changes you notice. Or try to work out on an empty stomach first thing in the morning, or experiment with a HIT approach. If fat-burning is your goal, avoid consuming anything but water for the duration of your exercise. Taking in sugary drinks, fruits, or other foods during exercise for a boost of energy will negate your fat-burning efforts, making your fat-burning zone "clock" back up or if a lot of calories are consumed, essentially reset, thereby requiring another significant period of time to burn through the consumed calories before burning fat. If you absolutely need to consume something, small pieces of fruit are low in calories and you will burn through them quickly, only setting you back 15-20 minutes or so in your fat-burning efforts. They can help give you a boost of energy to keep going longer, if an energy spike is something you require to get yourself into an effective fat-burning zone later on in the workout. Sometimes the small snack is well worth it to extend your exercise session into an efficient fat-burner. But, if you can plan ahead of time and eat an hour or two *before* the workout, powering through your entire session without having to take in any additional calories, you will likely be more efficient in attaining your goals.

When you are training for fat burning and are exercising first thing in the morning on an empty stomach, for example, do not expect to be as strong as you normally would be for weightlifting or other exceptionally physically demanding types of exercise. You are not going to set your personal best lift for squats or bench press on an empty stomach or at the tail end of a long workout, but you will be in an optimal fat-burning zone while hiking, running, cycling, walking, swimming, or doing whatever it is you find enjoyable. If you are determined to train on an empty stomach upon waking but find that you are hungry first thing in the morning, go ahead and eat something small. I know plenty of people who like to consume a piece of fruit first thing in the morning before starting their "fasted" cardiovascular training session. I often do the same. If I'm feeling hungry, I'll eat a banana and then get on with my workout. Even consuming water, which doesn't have any calories, sometimes tricks my mind into thinking I consumed something and I won't feel as hungry, and I can continue on doing whatever exercise I am doing that morning (often riding the stationary bike, wearing a hoodie, checking the morning news).

If 30-90 minutes sounds like an unrealistic amount of time to spend exercising, ask yourself what you are doing with the other 1300+ minutes in the day. Would spending an extra 30 minutes exercising to improve your health and fitness be time better spent than 30 minutes surfing the Internet or watching television, in relation to the goals you claim to care about? Finding excuses to skip exercise is easy, but the consequences of your priorities, revealed by your actions, are something you will have to embrace, come to terms with, or resolve to change. How badly do you want to succeed in your goals, and how can you improve your actions in ways that will support your mission? Answering these questions could be game-changers for your quality of health and fitness and perhaps for other aspects of life as well. Having an awareness of your level of activity, and your level of desire to manage your time appropriately to support your health ambitions are important, but so is knowing what to eat.

Fat-burning nutrition

A common understanding is that in order to burn fat, which is made up of approximately 3,500 calories stored in body, we must burn an excess of 3,500 calories more than we consume over a duration of time in order to lose one pound of fat. Though this can be done through strategic lifestyle planning, there are numerous factors involved, including the types of foods consumed, the rate of metabolism of the individual, level of exercise (which can impact the rate of metabolism), and ultimately the diligence of the individual to perform necessary actions required for fat burning on a consistent basis. Though a pound of fat in our bodies is approximately 3,500 calories, it takes about 4,000 fat calories consumed to put on a pound of fat. Where did the extra 500 calories go? Stored in our bodies, a pound of fat also contains water and protein, therefore not just pure fat calories, which would be closer to 4,000 calories. Ultimately this means it takes more calories consumed to put on a pound of fat than it takes calories burned to lose a pound of fat. This should be in our favor, right? As long as we adhere to consuming 10-15 percent of our total calories from fat, over a given time period sufficient for initiating results, having extra or unwanted body fat should be a non-issue, especially if we are exercising on a regular basis and avoid processed foods. But we all have different body fat percentage goals, different athletic and health goals, and different starting points. Knowing how to eat to reduce body fat is a valuable tool for anyone. For some it could be as simple as just eating exclusively whole, unprocessed foods with a total daily caloric percentage of 15 percent fats or lower to reduce body fat to a desired level. For others, it may be expending 500 calories more than consumption on a daily basis to burn an excess of 3,500 calories than consumed per week to drop a pound of body fat a week and lower overall body fat percentage. And yet for others, it may require a change in meal frequency and level of physical activity to change the rate of metabolism to work in the favor of effective fat burning. Though there are multiple ways of achieving your fat-loss goals, there are some common themes to help you get there. It starts with understanding the implications of eating various types of foods.

Some foods are healthier than others, some carbohydrates provide better fuel, and others are better for recovery. But some foods that the majority of the population eats are nutritionally void and do more harm than good. Avoid those foods. You know them; the processed, refined, sugar-laden foods that make us fat and cause a variety of illnesses. The following insight on carbohydrate selection will help you choose the right foods to fuel your athletic pursuits.

Simple carbohydrates such as table sugar, candy, soft drinks, maple syrup, and other sweeteners low in overall nutrition burn quickly, like newspaper on a fire. On the other hand, complex carbohydrates such as fruits and vegetables, grains such as oats and brown rice, and starches such as potatoes, yams, and beans, burn slower, like a log on a fire. It will take you much longer to burn through a meal of brown rice and beans versus a sugary snack. Cotton candy doesn't exactly stick with you for the long haul, unless we're referring to adding junk to your trunk, and not the good kind. Nor will crackers, chips, or vegan cookies provide you with healthy fuel. They might taste good but those foods won't help you achieve your goals, in fact, they'll inhibit your success. The fiber in the complex carbohydrates (whole foods) will help them burn longer, therefore fueling you longer. Some complex carbohydrate whole foods naturally have far more calories, and therefore more carbohydrates, than other foods. The upside of eating fruit right before exercise is that you will have a quick burst of energy, or fuel, that will burn out and turn into a fat-burning zone relatively early on in the exercise. The downside is that the energy will not be sustained very long, especially in comparison with potatoes, brown rice, or oats as fuel. The latter will give you energy for the long haul, but will also take a while to digest, process, and burn through to get into the fat burning zone (a full hour or more, depending on the caloric quantity, as well as the time of consumption in relation to time of exercise), whereas fruit calories could burn in half an hour or less.

Some foods will naturally be healthier, such as whole vegetables like sweet potatoes versus refined and processed pasta, for example, though both are common complex carbohydrate foods for athletes. Knowing how many calories per pound or per serving size for a given food could be helpful as well. Salad greens are only 100 calories per pound, for example; therefore, they would not be an ideal fuel source before a workout compared with sweet potatoes, which are 500 calories per pound, of mostly energy-producing carbohydrates. A pound of sweet potatoes would give you five times the calories, and due to the macronutrient make-up of the foods, likely more than five times the carbohydrates per serving. If consumed a couple of hours before exercise, some of the calories will have burned off during that time while still providing quality levels of energy to power through a workout. There are numerous websites that provide calorie counters and calculators that you can use to determine how many calories are in a given food. For example: www.caloriecount.about.com. Many people use MyFitnessPal to log calories consumed throughout the day as well (www.myfitnesspal.com). Others referred to me by some of my colleagues include www.loseit.com and www.cronometer.com. Regardless of which application you use, these are incredibly helpful resources to take the guesswork out of determining the caloric content of given foods.

The following is a general list of calories per pound found in popular foods, which I learned when completing the T. Colin Campbell Plant-Based Nutrition Certification Course through Cornell University.

Caloric Density of Food (approximate number of calories per pound from the following foods):

Healthy Foods

Salad = 100 calories per pound
Vegetables = 200 calories per pound
Fruits = 300 calories per pound
Starches (potatoes, rice, beans) = 500 calories per pound
Nuts and seeds = 2,000-2,500 calories per pound

Popular Foods

Cheese = 1,700 calories per pound
Chocolate = 1,800 calories per pound
Potato chips/fries = 2,500 calories per pound
Ice Cream = 3,000 calories per pound
Oil (pure fat) = 4,000 calories per pound

Does this list alone help explain where some of our excess bodyweight and body fat comes from? Simply becoming aware of information like this can give us a whole new perspective on what truly is healthy eating behavior. Clearly some foods should be avoided at all costs because they are directly linked to not only excess fat gain, but can contribute to a host of additional health problems. High cholesterol, high saturated fat, and animal-based foods are some of the leading causes of disease in the entire world and should be avoided in your quest for fat-loss, improved health, and more sustainable, compassionate living. Be transparently aware of your own food consumption too. We often give ourselves a pat on the back for eating a salad. What if a large bowl of salad, which should be just a few hundred calories, is covered in oil, which is how millions of people eat salad? It could turn into a 1,000-calorie meal made up of 70 percent fat. This happens to millions of people every day, and now the salad they are giving themselves a pat on the back for eating is actually more calorically dense than a burger or pizza and also contains more fat. It may not have the cholesterol and may not contain animal products like the burger or pizza, which I applaud from a compassionate perspective, but nutritionally, the salad covered in oil could be just as bad, or worse, than many common junk foods such as fast food and frozen dinners.

Given this information, and the list above, you can plan your meals accordingly. Eat starchy complex carbohydrates two to three hours before exercise so you can digest and start to burn through them. Or eat a faster burning complex carbohydrate like fruit within half an hour of exercising, knowing you will burn through it quickly and will move into a fat-burning zone in a short amount of time. Avoid simple carbohydrates (think soda and candy) because they are almost exclusively refined, processed, concentrated sugars that do not contain fiber. They are nutritionally void, contain concentrated calories, and are not healthy. Simple carbohydrates may be tempting due to their artificial flavors and addictive nature, but they only provide you with a quick burst of energy that will fade away early into your exercise routine, often in the first ten minutes or so. Additionally, they have numerous unhealthy side-effects such as excess fat gain and damage to dental health. They are also a waste of money and if you respect how hard you work to earn money, then there is no place for refined foods in your diet on a regular basis. Therefore, whole foods will always be your best choice for optimal fuel and health because they contain fiber, water, vitamins, minerals, proteins, carbohydrates, fats, amino acids, and other important nutrients. Stick with whole foods to carry you through your whole workout.

Putting principles into action

I was a competitive bodybuilder for a full decade, and this was my approach to burning fat: My regular bodyweight was around 180-185 pounds most days of the year. As I approached a bodybuilding competition six to twelve months in the future, I bulked up with muscle and fat to 195 pounds (using the muscle-building techniques I cover in the next chapter). As I got within three months of the competition, I started my fat-loss approach to reduce my weight from approximately 195 pounds to the competition requirement for the middleweight division of less than 176 pounds. *(The middleweight division includes bodybuilders weighing between 159 ¼ pounds and 176 pounds. I deliberately drop just below 176 pounds to be at the very top of the weight class. This is a strategy that works well for some bodybuilders and not very well for others due to numerous factors such as height and body type. It was my preferred approach to give myself the best opportunity to succeed by appearing to be as big as possible within my weight class).* Therefore, my objective was to drop at least 20 pounds while maintaining muscle and shredding unwanted fat, to reveal muscle size and definition on the bodybuilding stage. Essentially, I still wanted to look like I weighed 195 pounds, while in reality weighing 170-something pounds, but without the body fat that I had when bulking up. By getting incredibly lean, it can make muscles appear to be bigger than they are because muscle definition is revealed and is no longer hidden under layers of body fat. *This is what many magazine cover models do to make themselves look as good as possible, hanging onto muscle, while shredding the fat preparing for a photo shoot. Though it can be hard to sustain that kind of ripped physique year round, it certainly can be done if the right methods are followed with consistency.* As a semi-retired bodybuilder, that is one of my goals these days, to be in great shape year round. Eating whole foods day in and day out, I am fueling myself for exercise performance and don't have a yo-yo diet that most bodybuilders follow. Even in comparison to my previous competition years, now I don't have to jump from 195 to 175 pounds, but rather, I can stay at 185 pounds, or any other desired and comfortable body weight throughout the year while looking fit and muscular as a result of my whole food, 70/15/15 plant-based diet. For additional examples of bodybuilders who stay in great shape year round, check out Chad Byers, Derek Tresize, and Torre Washington, featured later on. These champion vegan bodybuilders stay lean year round and have incredible physiques because of their dedicated training and nutrition programs. This next example shows precisely how I effectively dropped 20+ pounds in a short amount of time by following methods that actually work. You can incorporate some of these same strategies to achieve your own fat loss goals.

This is the approach I followed to effectively burn fat and take my body from 195 pounds to as low as 171 pounds in 12 weeks or less, often in just eight weeks.

Four or five days a week I would wake up, and after brushing my teeth and drinking water (zero calories), immediately engage in low impact cardiovascular training for 25-45 minutes in a pure fat-burning zone. I rode a stationary bike, climbed on a stair-stepper, went for a hike, or climbed real stairs in a building at a moderate pace. If you're not a morning person, this can be a challenge. I am not a morning person because I keep very late nights, working on projects such as writing books, but because my goals were important to me I found ways to get to bed earlier, wake up with enthusiasm, and get my workouts completed. Often, turning on some of your favorite music in the morning helps get a little spring in your step to make it out the door to go sweat. Music or an internal dialogue recapping your goals in your own mind could be some helpful motivation to fuel your efforts.

Five days a week I would also lift weights. Therefore, at least four of five days I would do some fat-burning aerobic training in the morning *and* muscle building workouts at night, for a total of two workouts four days a week, with another day of just lifting and two full rest days. I lifted weights for approximately an hour and fifteen minutes in the early evening after a full day of eating healthy meals, focusing on training one or two muscle groups per workout (such as back and shoulders). Then I would again ride the bike, use the stair-stepper, or go for a hike, or jog immediately after weight training. This second round of cardiovascular training following my weight training workout often did not exceed twenty minutes. I would not eat anything during exercise to ensure an optimal fat-burning zone at the end of the workout. I took two days off per week to rest and recover and frequently used a steam room and sauna to help relax my muscles, and I stretched in those heated rooms to stay loose and help prevent injuries from having stiff or tight muscles. I focused my food consumption on unprocessed whole foods as often as possible to support fat-burning efforts. I ate a variety of plant-based whole foods, some processed foods, and used a few supplements. I recall one time going six weeks without consuming a single energy bar (which was a favorite snack of mine), because I wanted to avoid extra sugars and eat cleanly. Discipline was something I focused on and I routinely taught myself new levels of commitment. I competed as a bodybuilder eleven times in ten years and used this approach essentially every time. I always made weight, though there were a few close calls over the years, and I did well on the bodybuilding stage, winning multiple times and finishing runner-up four times.

Most competitive bodybuilders follow a similar approach to fat burning because it works. This approach is not just for bodybuilders, though. It is not a secret that only an exclusive group knows. It is a tried and true approach to reducing fat from your body. If you are willing to exercise on an empty stomach first thing in the morning, or engage in cardiovascular training after your primary workout is over, or will increase your intensity to get into a HIT zone, and will commit to eating healthy whole foods, fat-burning success is yours for the taking. Above all else, remember this. If you're willing to work incredibly hard in your athletic training, to the point that you train once or twice a day, four or five days a week, you owe it to yourself to eat the foods that will support your health and fitness goals. At the end of the day, one of the largest obstacles in the way of our goals is the fact that many of us exercise fairly regularly but are unwilling to reject animal-based and processed foods. Our results and our health suffer because of this. Exercise increases appetite, and avoiding succumbing to the desires to eat junk food (including common processed foods) is of paramount importance. If you do it right, you can exercise as much as you want and eat as much as you want, as long as the foods you eat are low on the calorie density scale such as leafy greens, fruits, vegetables, and starches such as potatoes, rice, and beans.

Respect the efforts of your precious time that you have committed to exercising by eating healthy plant-based whole foods. Get out there and shred it!

– CHAPTER 5 –

Building Muscle with Plants

> *"Fear is what stops you...courage is what keeps you going."*
> — Unknown (But I bet whoever first said this was totally awesome!)

P lant-based athletes consume adequate, quality protein on a pure plant-based diet and thrive with high levels of health and fitness. Building muscle by eating plants need not be considered a challenge, but viewed as an opportunity to show how beneficial it is to eat foods that contain the highest quality nutrition. Maybe a plant-based diet and vegan lifestyle weren't popular in the '80s or '90s, especially among athletes, but they are today. A growing number of weekend warriors and competitive and elite world-class athletes are all realizing a common truth; plants provide the best energy, the best recovery material, and the best nutrition available. To follow a plant-based diet as an athlete is to support your athletic endeavors, equipped with the best tools to achieve success. It's really not that complicated either. The foundational sources of nutrition, vitamins, minerals, proteins, fats, and carbohydrates, come in their original (and best) forms from whole plant foods. Only plants contain fiber. Plants are free from cholesterol. Plants contain on average sixty-four times more antioxidants than animal-based foods, and plants are quite literally nature's perfect foods.

Source: http://nutritionfacts.org/video/antioxidant-power-of-plant-foods-versus-animal-foods/

Getting enough calories and specifically enough protein in our diet to help build muscle is something many athletes concern themselves with. Some stress about this quest rather dramatically, consuming powders, bars, isolated nutrients, fortified foods, and whatever else they can to ensure they have enough of this revered nutrient in their diet to achieve their goals. If only they knew they didn't need as much protein as they think, they could save a lot of time, money, excess calories, and digestive issues by opting for more nutritionally balanced whole foods, high in complex carbohydrates. Their kidneys and waistlines would likely thank them too.

Adjusting your caloric intake in order to achieve muscle-building results comes down to knowing what to eat and when. Eat frequently, eat quality whole foods, and consume them in adequate quantity to elicit the kind of muscle gains you are looking to experience. Combine your sound nutrition approach with regular resistance weight training, keeping specific goals close in mind. Above all else, ensure that each of the aforementioned nutrition and training principles are followed with consistency, accountability, and transparency.

Ask yourself if you *really* exercise five days a week and have documentation of it, or if you are *guessing* that you probably train about five days a week, without any accurate records to confirm your postulation. Do you *really* have a solid whole-foods nutrition program, filled with fruits, vegetables, nuts, seeds, legumes, and whole grains, or do you *imagine* your diet is pretty healthy, without total awareness of what you are eating each day? Complete transparency will clearly show us how we can adjust our nutrition and training programs to improve upon them, supporting the goals we strive to achieve. What we do not know can hurt us. The more aware of our actions we are, the more control we have to change them for the better.

Just as in the case for fat burning, if building muscle is your goal, you must likewise learn how the process works before effectively achieving it. You cannot expect to pack on muscle without understanding the basic biochemistry of it. Questioning my own ability to build muscle is how my bodybuilding career began. For an entire year I tried to gain muscle, and the end result was gaining a single pound. However, as I learned more about the muscle building process, I was able to add nearly thirty pounds of muscle the following year, as I made the transition from runner to bodybuilder. Let's look at the basics to get a good understanding of why building muscle seems to come so easily for some, yet others struggle with the same task.

Muscle grows as a result of micro-tears that happen within a muscle during resistance exercise such as weight training. Lifting weights, and putting your body under physical stress in other ways (such as manual labor or bodyweight exercises), causes muscle fibers to tear. The ensuing nutrients we take in and the rest and recovery periods that follow, do the work of repairing and rebuilding muscle fibers, which results in new muscle growth. In general, multi-joint compound exercises yield the best muscle building results. These are exercises such as squats, bench press, deadlifts, pull-ups, lunges, leg presses, overhead presses, Olympic lifts, lifting and carrying heavy objects, and other power movements that require multiple joints (elbow and shoulder or knee and hip, for example) to be used in the exercise. Explosive multi-joint exercises such as throwing heavy items like sand bags or medicine balls work well, too. Slamming a sledge hammer onto an old tractor tire is a personal favorite for some, and a common exercise for many power and strength athletes. It is quite effective in stress-reduction as well. Creating a workout schedule consisting of compound exercises four or five days a week is a great approach to muscle building. This allows for two to three rest days per week following intense workouts. Since compound lifts such as deadlifts are so much more grueling for the body than say, bicep curls, you will need at least a couple days of rest per week for your body to recover, repair, and rebuild. After all, during rest after a workout is when muscle is actually built. You may know people who weight train six or seven days a week. I did the same for periods of time, but it isn't sustainable for a long time for everyone. Also, many people who train with weights six or seven days a week, train with lower levels of intensity compared to how I, and many other bodybuilders and strength athletes train. With the sheer volume of exercise, time invested, and effort put forth, rest days are all but required to make forward progress. Ego doesn't have a place in real weightlifting progress. Some see it as a weakness to take days off because training daily helps their ego, but it will also likely lead to injuries over time. In general, train for the results *you* are striving for, leave ego at the door, and gauge your own progress and alter your training program as desired based on results over time. If a muscle or entire muscle group is still significantly sore from a previous workout, it is a good rule to give it rest until the soreness subsides before training that same muscle or muscle group again. That is one way to gauge recovery. If you have mild soreness that is a regular by-product of consistent exercise, it may be okay to continue to train regularly, but significant soreness tells you your body is still repairing itself and to go train a different muscle group or to allow more rest time to fully recover.

In Chapter 9, I discuss repetition ranges, types of exercises and training styles, and list sample workouts to follow to build significant muscle. Now that we have covered some basic training methods to help you get on the road to effective muscle building, let's evaluate the nutritional requirements to support your training efforts.

For starters, you have a minimum caloric need just to maintain your weight, muscle, and health. This is determined by your gender, age, height, weight, and activity level (how many calories you are expending or *burning* each day). You burn calories in everything you do—from sleeping to eating to exercising—the more intense the activity, and the longer the duration of exercise, the more calories you burn. You clearly burn more calories by running than by walking when performed for the same duration. The same goes for working in a job that requires walking, lifting, and stair climbing versus one that involves sitting on a chair at a desk for the same length of time.

Due to the impact physical activity has on our caloric expenditure and nutritional needs, people who are physically active, including athletes and those with physically demanding jobs, burn far more calories than people who are generally inactive. Therefore, they require more caloric intake than their non-active counterparts to maintain weight and build muscle. The following information is one of the most important components in altering your physique and is not to be overlooked.

If there is one major take-away here, aside from the motivational messages throughout, this is it: You can understand your own daily caloric needs based on your lifestyle by using the Harris-Benedict Equation. This helps you determine your Basal Metabolic Rate (BMR), which enables you to know how many calories you need to consume to maintain weight and remain healthy even if you are inactive. Establishing your minimum daily requirements will give you a baseline from which to work. You can use this equation to determine the very basic caloric intake needed each day. Then, factoring in your activity level, which will include additional calories burned or expended, you can determine how many calories you will need to consume in order to gain weight (muscle), if that is your goal. Consistent exercise and proper nutrition will enable you to bulk up with muscle, while limiting gains in fat. This formula, of course, also helps us determine how many calories we need to consume in order to burn fat and drop weight, using the same principles of identifying true caloric intake versus caloric expenditure based on our actual individual metrics.

The Harris-Benedict Equation (English Formula):

Men: BMR = 66 + (6.23 x weight in pounds) + (12.7 x height in inches) – (6.8 x age in years)

Women: BMR = 655 + (4.35 x weight in pounds) + (4.7 x height in inches) – (4.7 x age in years)

For a thirty-year-old male with a height of five feet eleven inches and a bodyweight of 175 pounds, using this equation, his BMR would be 1,858. This represents the number of calories his body will burn daily if he is not engaged in any extra physical activity during the day. Burning nearly 2,000 calories per day without doing anything, gives us some sort of an idea of how much we need to eat in order to build muscle, especially if we are quite active during the day. The man in this example may burn an additional 1,858 calories just doing his day-to-day activities, including exercising, and therefore need to consume at least the number of calories he is expending, 3,716 (1,858 x 2 for this example), in order to build muscle.

For a thirty-year-old female with a height of five feet five inches and a bodyweight of 135 pounds, using this equation, her BMR would be 1,406. Again, this represents the number of calories she would burn throughout the day without being engaged in any extra physical activity.

The following formula is helpful in gauging how much one should consume based on activity level:

Exercise Level	Daily Calories Needed
Little to no exercise	BMR x 1.2
Light exercise (1-3 days per week)	BMR x 1.375
Moderate exercise (3-5 days per week)	BMR x 1.55
Heavy exercise (6-7 days per week)	BMR x 1.725
Very heavy exercise (twice per day, heavy workouts)	BMR x 1.9

You can use the equation above to find your own BMR, or you can find on-line calculators in which to input data to reveal your BMR score. Just search "Harris-Benedict Equation calculator" and you will find an easy method for doing so. Your BMR will change as you age and as your weight fluctuates, so it is a good idea to check your score every so often as your body changes. This could be every few months, once a year, or when you notice significant changes in bodyweight, for example. The Harris-Benedict Equation gives us a good starting point, but unfortunately, it does not take into account lean body mass (your body weight excluding fat). Therefore, it will project an estimated caloric intake for someone who weighs 200 pounds, whether they have 8 percent body fat or 28 percent body fat. The activity level table above helps sort through that and provides clarity, but there is still some gray area.

In general, leaner athletes will require more calories than less lean athletes. With a lower body fat percentage than an athlete of similar size, the leaner athlete will not have the fat stores to call upon and therefore must consume more calories throughout the day to feed and replenish their body than their less lean counterpart.

For example, let's evaluate this scenario: Bodybuilder X wants to build muscle. He doesn't keep track of his caloric intake but figures he's a big eater and guesses he consumes around 4,000 calories per day. He's a hard worker so he's in the gym once or even twice a day, burning a lot of calories. As a go-getter, he even goes out of his way to lift heavy things for fun. If there is an opportunity to carry a heavy bag, do some manual labor at home, or climb stairs for the fun of it just to build calf muscles, Bodybuilder X is on it. He's the kind of guy who takes pride and pleasure in carrying his bike rather than riding it. He's that cool. But here's the problem. Bodybuilder X sounds like a cool guy, pretty determined and poised for success, right? He would be if he had been aware, accountable, and transparent about his diet. He *thinks* he is eating a lot and eating well, but when put to the test and asked to reveal everything he eats each day for two weeks, he is exposed for not putting himself in a position to build muscle, despite his enthusiastic efforts. This is why Bodybuilder X was also asked to record his workouts for two weeks and his general activity level. When all the details were on the table, Bodybuilder X was actually burning 4,200 calories per day while only consuming 3,400 calories per day. This whole time he just *guessed* that he was eating a lot (and eating enough to achieve his goals) but the reality of the situation was revealed to show that he wasn't even eating the minimum number of calories to maintain weight! Will Bodybuilder X build any muscle with this enthusiastic approach, which includes the hardcore action of carrying his bike rather than riding it and multiple workouts per day? Nope. In fact, he is more likely to lose weight and burn fat because of his caloric expenditure to consumption ratio. Poor guy. He seemed so pumped up about his goals too. This scenario happens far too often. People are willing to work so hard and go out of their way to commute to the gym twice a day, buy all sorts of supplements, do extra laundry (gym clothes), stay up late from taking stimulating energy drinks, and perform all these additional tasks they put on their plate, in the name of building muscle or changing their physiques. But these same *committed* individuals won't bother to document their nutritional and training programs for full transparency and that single oversight can cost them their fitness goals and dreams.

If you're willing to do everything listed above, which takes significant time, energy, and money, but you're not willing to jot down your meals and workouts, that specific inaction could be preventing your progress without you even knowing it. Well, now you know. That is how significant this oversight is. It completely changes the fitness outcome for millions of people every year. Making this one alteration in your pursuit to a desired physique or desired level of health and fitness can make the difference.

If we objectively critique Bodybuilder X, we can notice that day in and day out he is eating roughly 800 calories fewer than he is expending. Though this figure will vary on days he is not working out, he is still on pace to actually lose about a pound per week, rather than gain any weight. To be fair, he could be burning a lot of fat, and possibly building an almost immeasurable amount of muscle from his hardcore training, but he is in a daily caloric deficit, so he is unlikely to reach his goals. Obviously, he will eventually run out of fat to effectively burn and will actually start to burn a bit of muscle with his athletic pursuit. If Bodybuilder X would cut down to training once per day rather than twice and get his caloric expenditure down to 3,500 per day, and increase his caloric intake by an easy 400 calories per day (a couple of large yams), he would be consuming 3,800 calories while only burning 3,500 on training days, likely closer to 3,000 on non-training days, and he'd be in an anabolic (growing) state, rather than a catabolic (shrinking) state. If Bodybuilder X continues to monitor these numbers every week, he can adjust them based on progress. Perhaps he ends up getting down to 3,200 calories expended per day while consuming 4,200 per day. If the calories come from whole foods (not fatty, refined, or sugary foods) he is very likely to gain muscle, not fat. And with a net caloric intake of 1,000 calories per day more than he is expending, in this scenario, he should be able to attain his goals of building muscle and proudly walk around his community carrying his bike with bigger biceps and stronger calves.

We know we need to eat well and eat often. But what we eat, and what we choose to not eat, are also important factors. It is a common practice for an athlete to consume 0.8-1.2 grams of protein per pound of bodyweight to maintain muscle, and even more to *build* muscle. This is a theory I followed for over a decade as a competitive bodybuilder. From the time I switched from being a runner to being a bodybuilder at age twenty, I added 40 pounds of muscle consuming a plant-based diet. I gained 75 pounds total after switching to a plant-based diet as a 120-pound teenager. That high protein approach to building muscle was a system I believed in until I came across the research of Dr. T. Colin Campbell, bestselling author of the book, *The China Study*, and one of the world's leading authorities in nutritional biochemistry. Known as perhaps the top nutritional scientist in the world today, he proposed some compelling arguments that left me reevaluating my approach to bodybuilding nutrition. Dr. Campbell was in the audience for the first lecture about plant-based health and fitness I ever gave, back in 2005 in Vancouver, Canada. I was somewhat familiar with his work but didn't pay much attention to it until I started working for the film, *Forks Over Knives*, in 2011, of which Dr. Campbell is the star. Working for the powerful and highly influential documentary, communicating with the producer, Brian Wendel, and entertaining some new ideas about sports nutrition, I became less enthusiastic about the high protein, high supplement, processed food diet that I had been following for some time. Of course I always ate plenty of whole foods, but the processed foods, supplements, and emphasis on high protein foods was always there and made up a significant portion of my caloric intake. By 2011, working in the *Forks Over Knives* office in Santa Monica, CA, I found myself touring on their behalf and sharing the same stage as Dr. Campbell. I introduced the film to audiences and hosted Q&A sessions with Dr. Campbell and others on an expert panel and I was starting to get on board with his way of thinking. When I enrolled in the Plant-Based Nutrition Certification Course through Cornell University in 2012 my diet shifted in a complete 180 degrees from what it was during my years of competitive bodybuilding. They say habits are hard to break, especially some we have been following our entire lives or our entire professional careers, but given the thought-provoking evidence in support of a whole-food diet I was presented with, as an objective free-thinking individual, I had no choice but to give it a try.

Dr. Campbell's research shows we need just 5-10 percent of our daily caloric intake in the form of protein. Not one gram or more per pound of bodyweight, which would be more like 20-25 percent (or more) of our total caloric intake, but simply 5-10 percent of total calories. Consuming 20-25 percent of total calories coming from protein is something many bodybuilders and other athletes do on a regular basis (and what many non-athletes do too). Some even aim for 50 percent of their calories coming from protein. Though high protein consumption will help build muscle, it comes with a price. The price is a costly one, with risks such as potential cancer tumor growth, formation and passing of kidney stones, kidney disease, general stress on the liver and kidneys, the formation of plaque along artery walls, the damaging of endothelial cells that protect our arteries, and an increased risk for many diseases including obesity, heart disease, and cancer. It also can come with numerous not-so-pleasant side effects such as bloating, gas, feeling heavy, lethargic, and full. Trouble sleeping due to the tough process of digesting all those dense calories is also a complaint among some followers of a high-protein diet. Though Dr. Campbell's research suggests animal protein is more likely than plant protein to lead to these adverse health conditions, many side-effects, including those listed above, can become present no matter what type of high-protein diet is consumed. I suffered many of these ill side effects for many years believing it was a sacrifice necessary for me to achieve my fitness goals while maintaining my compassionate vegan lifestyle. I'm glad I know now what I didn't know then, and I am pleased that I am able to share this refreshing perspective with others.

Reducing the amount of protein an athlete consumes is almost sacrilegious, and it garners ideas of fear of losing muscle and withering away. I assure you those outcomes do not have to come to fruition and I hope you are willing to give a lower protein, higher carbohydrate whole-food diet a try. Reducing the risks of serious health problems is enough motivation for most, and the curiosity to test a new theory will likely encourage other readers to get off the fence and eat from the garden.

To add some extra confidence to those who are leery about this transition, during the time of this writing, I recently gained ten pounds in ten weeks following an approximately 70/15/15 diet focused on plant-based whole foods. Though I have been following this exclusive whole-food diet since February 2013 and a mostly whole-food diet since May 2012, I started lifting weights after a six-month hiatus in early 2014, and muscle is coming back quickly as a result of consistency in both nutrition and training. A low protein diet has not inhibited my gains, and has actually allowed me to recover faster, have more overall energy, and build muscle while allowing me to be a better all-around athlete. Though I am in my mid-thirties, I feel as good as I remember feeling in my early twenties as far as energy levels and vitality. I routinely hear this sentiment echoed from others who transition to a healthy whole-food, plant-based diet, even if they were already on a vegan diet like the type I followed for a decade and a half before I adopted this new whole food approach. I enthusiastically encourage you to embrace this relatively low protein, 70/15/15 nutrition approach.

To put ourselves in a position to achieve our muscle building goals, we can simply follow the Harris-Benedict Equation to determine our BMR, and create a daily caloric plan accordingly. Then we can take that figure (say, 2,500 calories per day) and multiply it by five to ten percent, which would be our daily protein needs, and discover that we would need to consume approximately 125-250 calories from protein. There are four calories per gram of protein, so we would divide that number by four to get the number of grams, which in this case would range from 31.25 to 62.5 grams of protein per day. If you are a 175-pound athlete following conventional muscle building methods, you are likely consuming around 160-200 grams of protein daily.

Dr. Campbell's research, documented in *The China Study,* reveals that 5-10 percent of our calories coming from protein will *maintain* muscle. To *build* muscle, we need only increase our volume of food consumption beyond what we would normally eat to maintain weight, keeping our percentage of protein the same (five to ten percent). If we increase our total caloric intake to say, 3,000 calories, consuming the same macronutrient percentages as the original 2,500 calories, the amount of protein, which is synonymous with building muscle, will thereby also likely be increased (depending on the sources of the additional 500 calories), as will the amount of carbohydrates and fats—as all are macronutrients that make up food. The athlete we were just describing would now be consuming 150-300 calories from protein, which would be 37.5 to 75 grams of protein daily. This is an increase of 6.25-12.5 grams of protein per day, without changing the percentage of total calories coming from protein, with only a 17 percent increase in caloric intake.

You can see how easily you can adjust levels of protein, fat and carbohydrates simply by altering the volume of total calories. In fact, the challenge becomes avoiding eating too much protein, not the opposite, which is often emphasized as a concern by the general public for those following a plant-based diet. In today's western world (and all around the world, for that matter), most people would benefit from a reduction in protein consumption, and could still achieve their fitness goals by eating the right foods in the right ratios. For more strenuous sports such as weightlifting, football, mixed martial arts, triathlon training and so on, overall volume of food can be increased to meet the needs of the physical demand it takes to engage in those methods of training, especially if BMR is monitored through something like the Harris-Benedict Equation. Having a good understanding of your own caloric needs will clearly help you build muscle on a completely whole-food, plant-based diet.

You will find meal plans and recipes in the chapters to come that will be tailored to a sports-specific diet that features meal plans falling in line with the approximate amount of 10 percent of calories coming from protein, as well as others falling into a 70/15/15 category. It is unlikely that you will eat the exact same percentage of macronutrients daily, but having specific targets for meaningful reasons are good ideas.

The macronutrient percentage breakdown for an active person/athlete may look like this range, or somewhere within a few percentage points of each.

Percentage of calories

> 70-80% carbohydrates
> 5-15% protein
> 10-15% fats

Using a combination of low or high ends of these ranges can equate to 100 percent and give you a complete caloric breakdown of your daily food intake. You should also focus on consuming large amounts of water, because our muscles, brains, and bodies in general are made up of mostly water. Consuming half a gallon to a gallon a day for an active person is a good idea, aiming closer to the full gallon range. Some bodybuilders drink as much as two gallons of water a day to support their efforts. I have a small bladder so I drink what I can handle with my busy travel schedule on planes and in cars, but I believe most people, especially athletes, would benefit from drinking a gallon of water each day.

Exact macronutrient percentages may change daily based on diet, goals, lifestyle, and other factors (work, travel, and so on). In fact, it is unlikely that you will consume foods that naturally hit these exact percentages every day. Being absolutely precise is not the goal. In fact, that type of precision focus can lead to unnecessary added stress. The objective is to consume whole plant-based foods throughout the day that have macronutrient content that totals roughly those percentages outlined above. If you are within a few percentage points of any of those numbers, exercise regularly, and get adequate sleep, you are following healthy principles that will benefit your athletic endeavors, including building muscle.

These figures also vary by individual, based on factors such as your food preferences, your rate of metabolism, your specific athletic goals, and ultimately the types of foods you *actually* consume, not the ones you *think* you are eating. We tend to focus on the positive actions we take because we feel good about them and want to remember them, such as the times we have healthy meals or particularly good workouts, but we conveniently forget about the times we eat unhealthy food and do not exercise. We are often fooling ourselves in ways that will not support our goals. For example, you may strive to consume specific percentages of macronutrients, say 70 percent calories from carbohydrates, 15 percent from proteins and 15 percent from fats, but your actions could lead to something completely different, such as 40 percent calories from carbohydrates, 20 percent from protein and 40 percent from fat, which could easily happen when eating junk food at a party or a restaurant or bar. Are you *really* following healthy habits as consistently as you think you are? Remember, there are 52 weeks in a year, meaning there are 52 weekends, and if you consistently engage in poor health and exercise habits on weekends, you can see how that statistically becomes your *typical* behavior. When you add in holidays, birthdays, anniversaries, parties, travels, and other events, you could be looking at 50 percent of your days spent following poor health habits and you can imagine what impact this compounding effect has on your overall health. This reality is so much more important than many people acknowledge.

Being aware of your own behavior by documenting your food consumption for a week or two will give you incredibly helpful data from which to work in order to get closer to achieving your goals. The same accurate documentation is advised for your training regimen. Perhaps this alone will help you understand why you are building muscle, or why you are spinning your wheels. The same can be said for evaluating your fat-burning efforts. We already saw how Bodybuilder X struggled to meet his goals, and we found ways to remedy his situation to help him get on the right track to success.

Whether you are a professional athlete, weekend warrior, or consider lifting weights a hobby, building muscle on a plant-based diet should be easy, fun, and accessible regardless of where you are. Eat healthy foods, in large quantities if you are training regularly, and allow adaptation and muscle growth to happen. Be patient and understand that change takes time and that success is waiting for the determined, dedicated, and consistent athlete who puts in the effort day in and day out.

Have fun, stay motivated, visualize success down the road, and work hard consistently to achieve meaningful goals. Remember, if it is not fun, you likely won't do it. Find what inspires you, be consistent in your actions, and adaptation, improvement, and success are sure to follow.

As I emphasized in my book, *Vegan Bodybuilding & Fitness*, the most important thing you can do to support your health and fitness goals is to document your actual actions to be completely accountable and transparent about your exercise and nutrition programs. Doing so for a few weeks can be life changing. To ensure this is done, which increases the likelihood of health and fitness success, I am including new and improved training and nutrition journals for you to use as guidelines to create your own journals. You can also find 13-week training and nutrition journals on www.vegan-bodybuilding.com to track your actions and progress for months at a time. They will make a huge difference in your life. Simply having some sort of schedule and awareness of your true actions week by week will enable you to achieve true success, while understanding how you got there.

With these new and improved journals I am introducing the 3P. Or P to the power of 3:

Prepare – Perform – Produce Results

Workout Journal

Day _____ Date _____ Time _____

Pre-workout meal _____

Cardio workout _____

Warm-up _____

Workout Description _____

Exercise	Set 1 Weight/Reps	Set 2 Weight/Reps	Set 3 Weight/Reps	Set 4 Weight/Reps	Set 5 Weight/Reps

Post-workout meal _____

_____

Notes _____

_____

_____

Nutrition Journal

Day _____   Date _____

BMR based on Harris-Benedict Calculator _____

Total Daily Calorie Intake Goal _____

Macronutrient Ratio Goal (70/15/15) _____

Meal #	Time	Foods	Fluids	Calories	Totals

Notes _____

_____

_____

_____

– CHAPTER 6 –

Case Studies

> *"You don't set out to build a wall. You don't say, 'I'm going to build the biggest, baddest, greatest wall that's ever been built.' You don't start there. You say, 'I'm going to lay this brick as perfectly as a brick can be laid.' You do that every single day and soon you have a wall."*
>
> — Will Smith

I thought this quote was highly appropriate for a case study chapter because it exemplifies how success is created through small, deliberate actions; not by just saying, "I'm going to do something awesome. Watch me!" It's fine to make goals public and share them with others, but if you're constantly making claims and are not following through to achievement, perhaps your system and approach is broken and needs an intervention. Results are far more impressive and inspiring than making public announcements about all the great things you will achieve without matching the necessary action steps to support those desires, leaving them as unfinished projects and unattained visions. Making big, lofty, often out of reach goals to stroke our own ego won't get us far, but by hammering away at something meaningful, day after day, knowing that each action is one more step toward achievement, is the true road to success. One can still dream big, but the foundation must be built upon hard work and discipline, laying each brick one at a time in order to create the wall you desire.

Now that you have sufficiently learned about burning fat and building muscle in the previous chapters, let's examine some people who have done this effectively. My own experiences in burning fat and building muscle are the foundation upon which my entire career was built. Succeeding in those areas is quite literally how I built my business, my career, my reputation, and what truly enabled me to impact others, simply as a result of my actions and outcomes. It is through those actions that led me to be able to write this book with confidence, from decades of fitness experiences to draw from. Of course, there are plenty of amazing fat-loss and muscle-building case studies and transformation stories that far exceed anything I ever achieved, and I am honored to be able to share some of those stories with you. Get ready to be inspired by those who jumped into the action to make a dramatic change in their lives, rather than sitting on the fence wondering what might have been.

Being an athlete, there are always going to be ups and downs, and often injuries, setbacks, and other obstacles to try to juggle in life while still committing to maintaining high levels of fitness. I'll share a few examples of transformation from my experiences and I will enlist the involvement of some of my colleagues who have achieved outstanding results by following specific and deliberate actions that led to success.

I am a fan of case studies, of trial and error, and of failure and success. I talk openly about the times that I failed, the times I fell on my face, and the times I flat out hit the wall and had to start over. The reason I take pride in my failures is because I put myself out there so many times, and tried so hard to succeed, that I eventually did succeed in many areas of health and fitness that were very important to me. But I first had to fall down many times to pick myself up and learn from my failures to ensure the next time around would be more successful. Many people won't get out of the comfort of their own complacency to try to do something remarkable. Many people won't take responsibility for their own inaction and the shortcomings that follow. Many people won't own up to personal accountability and will find something or someone to blame around every turn. I didn't want to be one of those people and I was willing to try and willing to fail in order to learn how to succeed. You don't have to be one of those people either. You can choose to learn from failures and succeed to greater heights next time around.

This is an example of a personal case study of failure and success. Anyone who knows me knows that when I am passionate about something, I don't just go through the motions, I put the pedal to the metal and I crush it as hard as I can. I don't do things halfway, I go over the top. The same approach rang true with my bodybuilding career. I was a skinny farm kid who had no business in the sport of bodybuilding, especially as a vegan in the late '90s, but I embraced it and pursued it anyway. I wasn't supposed to succeed, but I did. But it also came with a price. I was never satisfied with the weights that I was lifting, knowing I was always capable of lifting more if I could just focus harder, believe in myself more, and find some way to push beyond barriers. This could be perceived as a motivating and uplifting approach to many reading this, or simply seen as obsessive compulsive or manic, but however you choose to perceive it, that approach, which helped me succeed, also left me injured more times than I care to remember. I pushed it so hard, often beyond the limits of what my 175-195 pound frame could handle. I was playing with fire and I was only partially aware of it, until I got burned too many times. After sustaining back-to-back painful injuries in my lower back and my wrist from being a little too enthusiastic with heavy weights in the gym, I decided to hang it up and retire from bodybuilding for a second time in 2012. The pain from the injuries and the physical limitations they left me with made it all too clear that enough was enough and that after a decade of pushing my body to the limit, I was done. At the ripe old age of 32, my bodybuilding career came to a sudden halt. I had already been on a hiatus from the competition stage from 2009-2012 as a result of releasing a book and touring, having some changes in interests, and you guessed it, another injury that I sustained in 2011. I was still active in the gym a few days a week during those years, but at a much more casual pace.

Prior to my injuries, in the early months of 2012, I had mounted another bodybuilding comeback. I was enthusiastic, consistent, driven, and poised to achieve perhaps my all-time best physique and new levels of bodybuilding success. I became strong again and was starting to put on some muscle, all on a whole-food, plant-based diet. I was hitting some record lifts, doing compound exercises I hadn't done in quite some time and I was progressing and enjoying the process. Bodybuilding, and weightlifting in general, was becoming fun again, perhaps the most fun it had ever been for me. Things were going well and I was excited about what the future would bring. A possible return to the bodybuilding stage, or maybe my best-ever physique, or more record lifts achieved. I was well on my way and everything was great. A few missteps in the gym left me down and out, and not just physically. When I sustained the back and wrist injuries in the spring of 2012, I took months off from the gym and I battled a depression I hadn't really experienced before. I stopped exercising all together, and didn't step foot in a gym for six months. I didn't even eat very much since I wasn't burning many calories and I got down to a bodyweight I hadn't been since I was a teenager more than a decade prior. I didn't look like a bodybuilder or a weight lifter or strength athlete, and I didn't want to associate with bodybuilding. I pursued some other interests in life such as casually studying Buddhism, meditating, traveling, and doing a whole lot of soul searching. I even left my apartment in Austin, TX for a few months as I drove out east to try to find myself. I set up a base in New England and sat on a few rocks by the ocean, by a river, or elsewhere and quietly looked inside to learn who I was at that time. I certainly wasn't the vegan bodybuilder everyone knew me as. I was a skinny shell of my former self, still recovering from injuries and unable to do anything about it, or so I thought. I turned down speaking gigs, rejected offers to be on TV, and to be interviewed for various publications, and I shunned the spotlight in favor of the darkness and quietness of internal self-discovery. I still wanted to be fit, but wasn't sure what to do. I almost had a sense of taking pleasure in watching my muscle mass disappear because it gave me an outlet to express my disassociation with the sport of bodybuilding and the lifestyle that left me in constant pain with deep frustration and resentment.

While on the east coast I met up with a fellow plant-based athlete, a vegan distance runner named Paul Mignosa who invited me to go for a run. I wasn't sure how my back would handle it, even though it had been a couple of months since I sustained my lower back injury. I joined him on a four-mile run in early August, which felt more like six miles and I was spent. My back was still sore and had to adjust to the stress of running. Like usual, I ran too fast, too hard, all too soon and I didn't run again for another week or more, as I was quite sore from the first outing and needed a significant recovery period. I know what you're thinking by now, what a stubborn guy this Robert character is. I would agree with you, but can assure you I'm working on being less assertive in exercise ambitions in favor of a more intelligent approach to training as I age. This is all part of a learning experience and I believe that as I age I become a little bit wiser.

I went on a few more runs with Paul in New England and then headed west. While back in Texas for a brief stint I learned of a three-hour timed trail race in Austin in December, ironically on my anniversary of becoming vegan, December 8. A friend encouraged me to sign up to run it, and I felt like it would be a good way to kick off my eighteenth year as a vegan athlete. I continued my training in Austin and then went to Oregon for the fall. When I made it back to Corvallis, where I'm from, I met up with an old running partner from my childhood. The friend who first introduced me to serious long distance running and who recruited me for the high school track and cross country teams, and later the Oregon State University cross country club, would be my training partner. Just like he did back in the '90s, Nick Martin pushed me and challenged me to become a better runner. We ran together regularly during the month of September and parts of October, and when he wasn't available to meet up, I ran on my own. I took a play out of my own book and followed a consistent training program knowing that it was leading to adaptation and that I was improving and that I would eventually succeed.

When I got back to Texas in late October, I prepared to run this race I had only been training for since early September. December 8 rolled around and my goal was to complete the race without having to walk. The week prior, I did a test run and only made it two hours, two minutes and two seconds before I had to call it a day. That was my longest training run in more than a decade and only a few runs during this training period lasted more than 90 minutes at a fairly fast, sustained pace. That is all the endurance I built up to in my short three months of preparation, after being injured for the majority of the spring and summer. Though I had only made it as far as two hours of continuous running up to this point, I had been consistent and over the past few months and I was able to run for that length of time at a swift pace, at least from my perspective, as a result of training and preparation.

Come race day, I only consumed fruit before the race, especially bananas, to give me easy digestible food that would provide quick energy, some prolonged energy, and would not be heavy on my stomach during my three hour pursuit to complete the race without having to walk. Though that was my goal—to finish the race without having to stop and walk—I did leave myself an out by having a bag filled with snacks, an extra pair of socks to change into, other clothes and even another pair of shoes, should I need them. I was prepared to stop and walk if need be, was prepared to eat and change clothes, was prepared to have fun, and was prepared for the challenge I had in front of me.

The course was a 1km loop (1,000 meters) through the woods on a winding trail that made it impossible to see more than 100 meters in front of you at any given time. Despite the temperature reaching 85 degrees on this December morning, I was in full form, in a rhythm, and I was immediately reminded of my competitive running days more than a decade prior within the early moments of the first lap. All of a sudden I was in my comfort zone in the midst of competing in a sport that had been foreign to me for the past third of my life. I felt amazing during the race and after an hour of going out much faster than planned (surprised?), I realized I was very likely in the top ten, as I was already lapping a bunch of other runners. After two hours, I realized I was in the top five, perhaps even higher. At this point I was in a lot of pain and could barely keep my eyes open, but I told myself over and over in my head, *Just keep running*. Not *Just keep going*, but very precisely, *Just keep running*. With approximately five minutes left, I learned I was in second place (feedback from a friend who was on the sidelines cheering and following our progress online through a digital chip we all had attached to

Shred It!

our shoelaces, providing real time updates online). I had already begun my kick before the final lap, figuring I was closing in on the leader, though I couldn't see him, and given the information that I was not far behind him, I turned it into a full sprint for the entire last lap. I was averaging about five minutes per lap and I knew if I had any chance of catching the leader, this would have to be by far my best lap. And there was nothing to lose. I was already in pain, I was already suffering, and with the end of the race looming just minutes away, I knew exactly what I needed to do to finish the story I had been telling myself in my head for nearly three hours covering more than 37 laps.

With my fastest pace of the entire race, I made up two full minutes on the final lap to catch and pass the leader just before the finish line. I won the race by eight seconds and set a new course record. It wasn't until after the race I learned that when I started my final lap I was two minutes behind the leader, who likely figured he was coasting in for the win (and the new course record). But I somehow ran that final 1,000 meters in a full-on, all-out sprint, with my eyes barely open, rolling my ankles through the loose bark mulch trail, flying past other runners as I lapped them with the most epic pursuit I have ever had in any race to get to the finish line. Because I finished a couple of minutes before the three hour mark, I ran an additional lap at full speed unaware of when the race was really over, when I had crossed the finish line minutes before the three hour mark or when the clock struck three hours. In case the leader I had passed tried to catch up and pass me to regain the lead, I just kept running. As it turns out, I had already won the race and the extra lap was unnecessary, but it added another half mile to my total, making it my all-time longest run in a single day of 22.5 miles. The official results list my course record at 21.749 miles, which was completed in around 2 hours and 57 minutes. The record still stands today, at the time of this writing in 2014, and I would be honored if it stands for some time, but I suspect it is temporary as there are far better runners than me out there. The winding trail with likely thirty turns every kilometer loop made it hard to ever get an even pace going and the rough terrain, and the narrow trail crowded with runners made it all the more challenging. By the end, I was exhausted from three hours of saying, "Passing on your left."

If we were to race again, I am fairly confident the runner who came in second would win nine out of ten times. I had no business running that entire race without stopping at the pace at which I ran, and had no business winning, but I did. I succeeded because I was able to find meaning in my training, because I fully understood how consistency leads to adaptation and improvement, and even though I only had a few months to prepare, I aimed for the best return on investment from my training by running with a champion runner and holding myself accountable by training hard when I was on my own. The real reason I won on that day, and likely would not win on any other day, was because I had a psychological advantage over everyone else on the course. It was my anniversary of becoming vegan, nearly two decades after making a decision that changed my life forever, and which forever guided my future decisions. I won that race because of the unbelievable willpower I was able to find within myself to be able to create the result to tell this story. I wasn't running just for myself, I was running and suffering with the pain I endured to acknowledge, honor, and respect the pain that innocent animals are subjected to in order to serve the interests of many humans. I chose to stand against that and to be the best runner on that day and to let it be known that no animals had to die for me to excel, achieve, and succeed as an athlete.

Though I probably wouldn't win if the stakes were different and not so perfectly positioned in my favor, I believe that we can harness that kind of energy and drive and create a psychological advantage in athletics even on non-anniversary days, on days that don't have any special significance in our lives. I believe we can mentally prepare ourselves for excellence if we can block out the noise of everyday distractions and tap in to the quietness of meaningful focus, intent, and a winning mindset. Therefore, I could recreate that outcome, and in fact, I have, with two great races in recent months. The inner strength was there all along. I just had to find it.

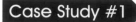

Case Study #1

A Vegan Bodybuilding
Transformation

By Derek Tresize

VeganMuscleandFitness.com

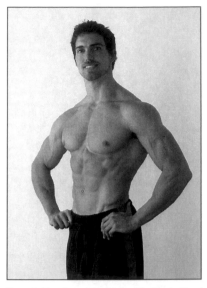

Derek Tresize - Photo by Kimberly Frost

Many find it hard to believe I have ever had a hard time gaining muscle from working out in the gym. I've had some success in natural bodybuilding competitions, earning first place in two, and there is already a misconception that anyone with muscle must have come by it through genetics. While I *have* taken naturally to weight training, which I started my first year of high school, I can honestly say all the gains I've made have come from consistent hard work, intense effort, and strategic planning of my diet and exercise regimens. I have always had a very fast metabolism so, while staying lean has never been a struggle for me, gaining muscle definitely has. When I became vegan in 2007, I weighed about 180 pounds at five foot eleven, with a body fat level of roughly 12 percent. After transitioning to a vegan diet that year, my already fast metabolism got even faster and I dropped to 170 pounds and 7 percent body fat with no additional effort whatsoever. While this was an exciting turn of events, I've spent most of my years in the gym trying to *gain* weight, not lose it, so my new, even faster, metabolism was a bit daunting when I considered my goals of gaining muscle mass and (someday) competing as a bodybuilder on stage. I maintained that weight and body fat for several years while I pursued martial arts and my weightlifting took a backseat. Then, in the fall of 2009 I was scheduled for my first ever physique photo shoot. I was in great condition and had very little work to do to prepare, but afterwards the photographer asked if I'd like to do another shoot in three months, and I decided that I wanted to gain as much muscle mass as I possibly could for the second shoot.

I hit the drawing board and wrote myself an intense training regimen that involved working out twice a day most days, and centering my workouts on heavy compound barbell exercises such as squats, deadlifts, power cleans, and presses. For my diet, I searched the web looking for some sort of vegan weight-gainer shake I could use to easily increase my caloric intake, and when I couldn't find one I decided to create my own. After some trial and error, my bean shake was born! In it I used white beans, oats, bananas, soy milk, seeds, and any other fruits or vegetable I could get my hands on to make a tasty smoothie that added over 1,000 calories to my daily diet. While I wouldn't recommend that big of a caloric surplus for most people, my fast metabolism took it in stride and I made unprecedented gains in the gym and on the scale. When I arrived at the photo shoot three months later, I was up about 15 pounds to 185 at around 6 percent body fat. I'd also gained significant amounts of strength, so I considered my experiment in vegan muscle gain a huge success, and the photos from that shoot rapidly spread across the Internet and were even featured in the local newspaper.

I've since gone on to compete in five natural bodybuilding competitions, two of which I placed first. In the summer of 2014, I entered my first physique competition and not only won first place but earned my professional status within the organization. I've also had a lot of success helping my personal training clients gain muscle and strength by incorporating whole plant foods and heavy barbell training into their fitness programs, so I know *my* results weren't exceptional. By focusing on the most health-promoting, nutrient-dense foods on the planet, getting plenty of calories, and training hard and smart, virtually anyone can add lots of muscle mass to their frame without compromising their health, ethics, or the environment.

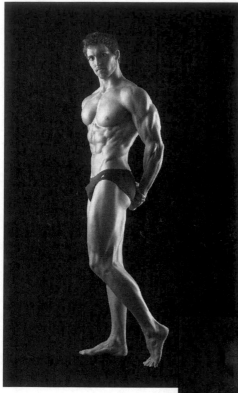

Derek Tresize
Photo by Kimberly Frost

Derek Tresize
and Marcella Torres
Photo by Kimberly Frost

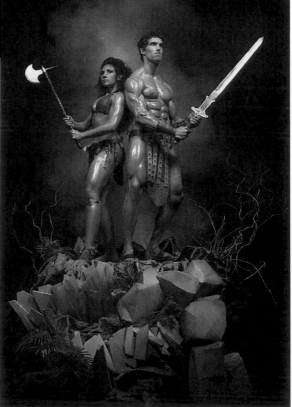

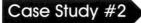

Case Study #2

A Vegan Body Revolution

By Thomas Tadlock

VeganBodyRevolution.com

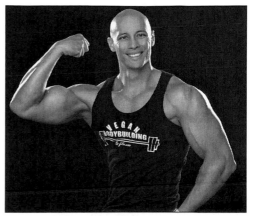

Thomas Tadlock
Photo by Melissa Schwartz
theveganrevolution.net

It took me nearly two years and five attempts to figure out how to build muscle on a vegan diet, using a whole-foods approach. In the first attempt, I simply tried doing my typical muscle building routine that I always followed successfully when I used to eat meat. I would train each muscle group once a week, and eat five to six meals a day. I tried consuming about one gram of protein per pound of bodyweight a day, which made up about 30 percent of my calories. Then I ate about 55 percent of my calories from carbohydrates, and the remaining 15 percent from fat. Only this time, I swapped out the meat with lots of processed vegan veggie hot dogs, nuggets, and burgers. It was an utter failure. I got fatter and weaker. My blood pressure and resting heart rates began to rise, and my energy levels dropped.

In my second attempt, I followed "The Meatless Machine II" plan that was in Tim Ferriss' book, *The 4-Hour Body*. I needed to modify that plan slightly so that it didn't contain any animal products. But sadly, after 28 days, I had virtually zero muscle or strength gains to show for it. Four months into being vegan, watching my physique degrade, I began to feel frustrated.

In my third attempt, I tried to combine the nutrition strategy that I read in vegan bodybuilder, Robert Cheeke's book, *Vegan Bodybuilding & Fitness* and the Colorado Experiment workout that's featured in Ferriss' *The 4-Hour Body*. The Colorado Experiment was a piece in Ferriss' book that featured a bodybuilder who gained an incredible amount of muscle in 28 days, much more than what is typically expected during that period of time. My thought was to copy the workout routine, while doing Cheeke's meal plan. For some reason, I couldn't seem to get it right. After 28 days, I gained two total pounds and just a little bit of strength. I was definitely doing something wrong. There must have been something I was missing. Maybe I misread the guidelines in Cheeke's book, or maybe I should have followed his workout plan.

It wasn't until the fourth attempt that I finally built muscle, but it wasn't from a completely whole-foods approach. I decided to increase my protein intake to 1.25–1.5 grams per pound of body weight, using mostly tofu, seitan, and pea protein powder. Plus, after reading many articles about vegan athletes' endurance and recovery improvements, I decided to double the volume of my workouts, doing twice as many sets for each exercise.

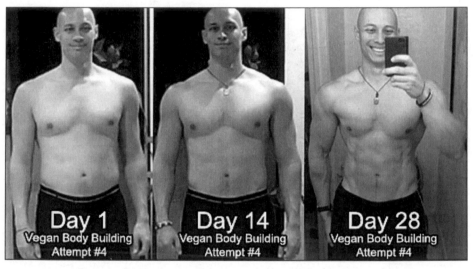

Thomas Tadlock - Before, during and after transformation

This attempt worked, and the results amazed me. Check out the progression pictures.

Although I achieved great results, and finally gained some muscle on a vegan diet, the diet and workout routine were complicated and filled with way more processed vegan protein powder than I was comfortable eating. I began searching for a better way to build a lot of muscle on a vegan diet.

Years later, I launched the Vegan Body Revolution Show podcast on iTunes so I could study the nutrition and workout programs of the top vegan bodybuilders in the world by having them as guests. After interviewing over ten of the top male and female vegan strength athletes in the world, having them share their day-by-day workout and meal plans, I experimented with a drastically different approach and did a fifth attempt. The fifth attempt was my most successful, which built even more muscle and I gained 10.1 pounds in 28 days.

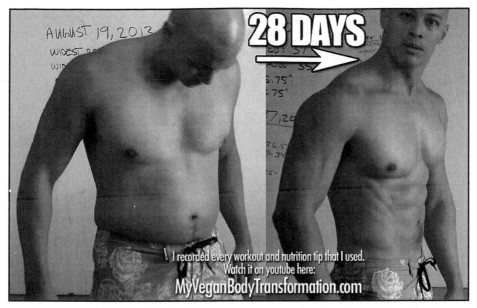

Thomas Tadlock - Before and after

Shortly after the success of my last vegan muscle-building attempt, I met a professional bodybuilder who made me doubt every belief I ever had about protein. I met Torre "Tha Vegan Dread" Washington at the Vegan Health & Fitness Magazine Expo in Los Angeles, CA. I was standing with my wife next to a stage where professional photographers were shooting photos of fit vegans. I had my back turned to the stage, talking with my wife, when I noticed her eyes bulge out of her skull. I turned around to see what she was reacting to, and then my eyes bulged out of my skull. Behind me was the most ripped and massive vegan man standing there shirtless with long dreadlocks.

I quickly introduced myself to Torre and we hit it off immediately. He turned out to be the nicest, most humble guy. We talked training and nutrition, and then we got to the topic of protein. What he told me blew me away. Torre stands at five-feet-seven inches in a compact muscle machine and weighs around 170 pounds. He consumes between 110 to 160 grams of protein a day. That's far less protein than what I was consuming on my last successful muscle building attempt, and the idea of eating less protein and getting just as massive really intrigued me. I thought this could be something worth experimenting with in the future.

Shortly after meeting Torre, I met another incredible vegan athlete who took first place in the fit model category of the 2012 Naturally Fit Supershow in Austin, TX, Chad Byers. Chad has a physique that makes your jaw drop from every angle. It's as close to a perfect physique as you can get by Men's Health magazine standards. Chad's most distinguishing feature is his massive arms. After interviewing Chad about how he built those arms on a vegan diet, he revealed something to me that made me flip out. What he told me went against everything I ever thought I knew about building muscle. He told me that he built and maintained his massively muscular physique eating only three meals a day. *Are you kidding me*? It was true. He showed me what he was eating. It turned out that he was getting the equivalent of six or more meals a day squeezed into three gigantic ones.

It took a little research, but I did, in fact, find some research studies that showed you could build and maintain muscle consuming only three meals a day. Chad was a living, breathing, super-ripped, massive example.

What I learned from Torre and Chad turned my whole paradigm of vegan bodybuilding nutrition upside down. It made me very curious about the possibilities of using less protein and fewer meals. What if it was possible to gain muscle without having to eat as much protein as a typical bodybuilding nutrition plan would recommend, and with half the meals? This alone could make it far more accessible for anyone, especially the busy family man or the woman who has too much going in her day to prepare six meals each day and carry them everywhere. My brain began obsessing, and I began a period of being a mad scientist to experiment with and explore the possibilities of making vegan muscle building easy.

Chad gave me an idea for the ultimate busy person's muscle building meal plan using three meals a day. Building muscle on three meals a day would be a real game-changer for so many people, so I created a three meal-a-day muscle-building plan. Going along with the theme of making vegan bodybuilding nutrition easier to do, I thought about how I could also simplify weight training. The traditional bodybuilding weight training routines that I have been taught involve myriad of exercises for each muscle group. Typically, it involves doing two to four different exercises for each major muscle group, performing three to four sets, and eight to twelve reps each. Focus on one or two muscle groups at a time, and train them once or twice a week. Those workouts were way too complicated. I needed to simplify them, so I did. I came up with a simple, four-exercise workout plan and put it to the test. I used myself as a test subject and applied my three meal-a-day, four-exercise vegan bodybuilding plan to myself over the course of four weeks and filmed every single workout. You can watch them on www.MyVeganBodyTransformation.com.

Do you know what happened?

I gained 10.1 pounds, 1.25 inches on each arm, shrunk my waist, and nearly doubled the weight in all of my lifts in the easiest, no stress way I have ever experienced. This was the easiest body transformation experience I have ever had. I believe simple is doable, and what's doable gets results. Below are the three key steps that I used to apply this fast and easy vegan muscle building system.

Step 1: I Ate Three Vegan Muscle-Building Meals A Day

Instead of eating five to six meals a day, I ate three gigantic whole food meals a day. This fit my busy family and travel lifestyle so much better.

Since I was only getting three meals in a day, I made sure that those meals were packed with as many nutrients as possible. In order to accomplish this, my meals consisted of almost nothing but whole foods and I ate to painful fullness every meal. Now, as a guy who loves to eat, I didn't mind this one bit.

Here is a small list of some of the whole foods that I eat mainly raw to get maximum nutrient value out of:

- Broccoli
- Kale
- Pluots
- Bananas
- Apples
- Tomatoes
- Avocados

I know that this list may seem very small, and it is. But really, this represented about 80 percent of everything that I ate during those twenty-eight days, and it worked beautifully. I bought these ingredients in bulk. I purchased bananas and tomatoes by the case and saved a lot of money.

I put these ingredients in a blender and made gigantic smoothies out of them, which I would drink 64 ounces of at a time. Here's an example of what I ate in one day. Keep in mind that I never counted the amounts of each food. I simply ate them to absolute painful fullness:

Meal 1 Summary

> 64 oz. Smoothie
>
> Lots and lots of watermelon

Meal 2 Summary

> 64 oz. Smoothie
>
> Veggie burger sandwich
>
> Quarter of hummus sandwich
>
> Some tomatoes
>
> Some apples
>
> Some plums

Meal 3 Summary

> 64 oz. Smoothie
>
> Huge flaxseed cracker
>
> Lots of frozen bananas

What about the protein?

One of the ideas I was testing is one that comes from Dr. Doug Graham and Dr. Caldwell Esselstyn, among many others (including Dr. T. Colin Campbell). They claim that your body only needs 5 percent to 10 percent of its calories from protein in order to build muscle. Taking all of the amino acids that come from eating the ingredients listed above to uncomfortable fullness yielded about 50 grams of protein a day for me. I sometimes added one to three scoops of rice protein powder a day to my diet, making protein shakes as a muscle insurance policy, which made my total protein intake come out to be about 65 to 98 grams a day. For a 200-pound guy like me, that's less than half of what the traditional bodybuilding guidelines would recommend.

I can't tell you *why* it worked, but I can definitely say that after becoming 10 pounds heavier and twice as strong, it worked.

Step 2: I Used Four Muscle-Building Exercises

To simplify the exercise component of building muscle fast on my vegan diet, I painstakingly studied the biggest physiques of all time. I studied their workout routines. I also studied the athletes who seemed to get the biggest the fastest, without "trying" to be a bodybuilder. What I noticed was power-lifters and football players are by far the biggest group of non-bodybuilder athletes. A powerlifter's sole focus is lifting as much weight as possible. A football player's focus is to be able to access maximum strength, while being in a state of fatigue. What I found very intriguing was that both powerlifters and football players do the same lifts. They focus on three basic movements: squats, deadlifts, and presses.

Then it started to make sense. These athletes are building massive muscles doing just three different exercises. Squats built the legs, deadlifts built the erectors of the spine, and presses built the arms, chest, and shoulders. If I added rows as a fourth movement that built the lats and scapula retractors, then we'd have a complete muscle-building program with just four exercises.

Traditional bodybuilding routines recommend three to four sets of three to four exercises for each body part, once or twice a week. What if I simply did nine to sixteen sets of one exercise for each body part, up to four times a week? It was worth a shot. The simplicity and elegance of this idea was just too appealing.

After four weeks, I nearly doubled the weight of nearly every lift. In fact, it worked better than any of the traditional, multi-exercise approaches I ever tried.

Step 3: I Trained the Whole Muscle

The biggest factor I've seen that slows the progress of gym-goers who aspire to put on more muscle fast, is that they're only working a portion of their muscles. Every skeletal muscle (the muscles that move your limbs), is comprised of three categories of muscle fiber types: red, pink, and white.

Here's an interesting tip I discovered about building muscle:

Muscle fiber types need to be trained very differently in order to grow!

- Red muscle fibers grow when you train to muscle failure with 20 to 40 reps

- Pink muscle fibers grow when you train to muscle failure with 6 to 15 reps

- White muscle fibers grow when you train to muscle failure with 1 to 5 reps

Your genetics determine how much of each muscle fiber type you have in each skeletal muscle. How many bodybuilding articles have you read that suggest a rep range of 8 to 12 for maximum hypertrophy (muscle growth)? People who were born with more pink muscle fibers in their muscles are the ones who will get the best results training in that popular rep range. That's not me, and it's probably not you either. In order to grow muscles, even if you've been skinny and scrawny like me all your life, you need to train all the muscle fiber types. Pyramids and drop sets are two of my favorite strategies for training all the muscle fiber types with a single exercise.

Pyramids

An example of a pyramid chest workout would involve using a bench press and starting with the highest weight that forced me to quit between 20 and 30 reps. I then increased the weight by 20 pounds every consecutive set, banging out as many reps as I possibly could. I kept doing this until I got to a weight that forced me to quit after two or three reps. Then, I took off 20 pounds after each consecutive set and continued to pump out as many reps as possible until I came back to my starting weight. That was a complete pyramid and thoroughly trained all the muscle fiber types in my chest. I used the pyramid strategy for all four lifts.

Drop Sets

An example of a drop set for my biceps would be using the heaviest weight possible for two to five repetitions of a biceps cable curl. Then, after reaching muscle failure, I immediately decreased the weight by one to two plates and grinded out as many reps as I could. Once I reached muscle failure again, I decreased the weight and immediately repeated the whole process again as many times as I could. The number of sets I did depended on how much pain I was willing to take at the time. There were training sessions where the burning in my muscles was so bad that I had to use the breathing techniques I learned at my wife's birthing classes to help get me through them. My drop sets typically went for about five sets. I continued until I had reached a total of 20 to 30 repetitions so I knew that I had trained all of my muscle fiber types.

Conclusion

No matter what method you use from this book to build muscle on a vegan diet, you will be able to improve the size and strength of your muscles, but you'll also better your health and help the planet at the same time. I wish you massive success and hope you enjoy the rewards of going vegan and building a strong, muscular body at the same time.

Get shredded on a vegan diet, my friend! Letting the world know how you got your amazing body is the ultimate form of vegan activism.

Case Study Summary

In both Derek's and Thomas's case studies of experiments conducted on themselves, you can easily notice numerous similarities. Though they had slightly different approaches, they had similar objectives, which called for some actions that mirrored one another, though they came to these conclusions on their own, years apart. They both started with fairly skinny frames, wanting to build muscle and bulk up on a vegan diet. Through trial and error, they both found that using compound, multi-joint weight training exercises like squats, deadlifts, presses, and Olympic lifts combined with a high calorie diet will get the job done. Not surprising, I found the same results to be true when I put on 40 pounds of muscle in a few short years in my early twenties. Heavy barbell and dumbbell exercises with a high caloric consumption in excess of your daily expenditure will almost always certainly produce muscle-building results. Though their approaches were similar, I think the most value comes from looking at their differences. Although not mentioned here, Derek has been known for his weightlifting style of completing five sets of five reps per exercise, aptly named the 5 x 5 approach. Thomas, on the other hand, decided to incorporate pyramids and drop sets in order to achieve high, low, and mid-range repetitions for just a few total exercises. Furthermore, I tend to focus on the eight to twelve repetition range for various compound multi-joint exercises that I believe will give me the greatest return on investment, and I also focus on exercises I actually enjoy, knowing that if the exercise isn't fun, I will have a hard time doing it. The more I enjoy the exercise, the harder I will likely push myself as well.

All of our approaches worked for the short term for our personally conducted experiments on our own bodies to achieve desired results (burning fat and building muscle). Each of our approaches also worked for the long term, as all of us have built our bodies, our reputations, and careers based on the hard work we were willing to put ourselves through, using methods that yielded positive results. Given our various approaches to succeeding in record-setting and championship fashion, I can't help but believe that there are some positive lessons to be learned here. It doesn't mean it will work every time, but staying focused on consistency and hard work while having fun can help you build a championship bodybuilding physique or whatever physique outcome you desire. Not to be overlooked is the elephant in the room with regard to *why* we succeeded. There is no question in my mind that at the core of why we were able to attain specific desired outcomes is because we all had clear goals, with meaningful reasons behind them that had timelines and deliberate action steps that supported our end results. Having a clear objective to work toward every day can make all the difference, as it did for us.

You might have to put your own body through various tests to find your ultimate destination. By reading these case studies, my hope is that you will find helpful strategies from each of our examples and incorporate the aspects that work best for you. If you don't want to add a 1,000-calorie bean shake every day, you don't have to. If you're not willing to drink a half gallon smoothie until you're painfully full, you don't have to do that either. If you don't want to run so hard you can barely keep your eyes open, or lift weights with so much effort you feel like you're in Lamaze class, that doesn't have to be part of your lifestyle. What you can do is realize what your own BMR is, what foods and exercises you truly like most, and develop an approach to health and fitness that will meet your specific goals.

Whether you follow one of our approaches in this chapter, or one of the following approaches in the next chapter, or learn valuable life-changing lessons from one of the chapters to come, make it a point to fully understand what your ultimate goals are, identify why they matter to you, and pursue them with as much enthusiasm as you can gather. You have 1,440 minutes each day to make your dreams happen, to write your own case study, and to create your own transformation. What are you made of?

– CHAPTER 7 –

Transformation Stories

> *"If you want to live a happy life, tie it to a goal, not to people or things."*
>
> — Albert Einstein

T here are few methods of grabbing someone's attention that are more effective than a powerful transformation. Whether we're talking about a dramatic physical transformation of someone who lost significant weight and completely altered their physique and changed their life, or a rags to riches financial transformation, a significant shift in where we were to where we are commands attention. Using this attention for positive influence is very noble and gives you a unique power to create change. I'm not talking about bragging and gloating. I'm talking about working your butt off for something you care about, and being a living example of positive transformation.

Transformation stories have always inspired me. I have been motivated by the hard work, sacrifice, and dedication others have endured in order to achieve something remarkable, especially in athletics. Like when I was a kid, hearing about Ozzie Smith using a brown paper bag as a baseball mitt because that is all he could afford at the time, and then going on to become one of the greatest players to play the game of baseball. Of course, the classic tale of Michael Jordan getting cut from his high school basketball team, only to become the most iconic and arguably best basketball player in history is another story many of us are familiar with. What about Mary Decker Slaney who competed in three Olympic Games and was one of America's most decorated runners for decades, even after multiple setbacks, including getting tripped and falling in an Olympic race, and having to be carried off in a stretcher? And who can forget America's greatest running legend, Steve Prefontaine, who wasn't necessarily built for running, but who willed himself to be one of the strongest and most dynamic runners to walk the earth, setting record after record during his short life? More recently, wrestler Anthony Robles, won the NCAA championship for his weight class despite only having one leg. He was the best wrestler in the entire country, never even losing a match his senior year, overcoming an obstacle that would keep many people off the mat and on the sidelines. Tennis player, Serena Williams, won 78 of 82 matches in 2013 after changing her diet to a plant-based one to support her sister, Venus, the world's former #1 player, who adopted a plant-based diet to help overcome health issues.

These examples, and countless others, serve as motivation for many of us. This is what moves us and makes us want to go out and practice what we love, to improve and become champions ourselves. It is what helplessly compels us to run stairs, throw the football, or shoot baskets until midnight, believing we too can become remarkable. Or perhaps it inspires us to go out for a run, head to the gym, or go outside with a soccer ball and hone in on our own craft, practicing, determined to get better because we were inspired by stories of those who put in the time to get where they were going.

Physique transformations are the ones we are focusing on in this book. There are many people in the plant-based athlete community who have inspired me and plenty of others, who have made a name for themselves, simply from leading by example. When you walk your talk you don't really even have to say anything. Your actions speak for themselves and you naturally become a leader in your community. There are many outstanding individuals who have been flying under the radar for a while, and I feel very fortunate to have met a number of them on tour, or to have stumbled upon them online, to be able to invite them to share their story with you. Some are unassuming, quietly going about their business, and do not have a strong presence online or an extroverted personality, but they spread a positive message and lead by example through their actions.

As I did with the case studies, I'll begin with my own transformation. You read about some of my transformations from my early days of bodybuilding, but you probably don't know about this, more recent transformation:

My physique transformation—2013

When I was asked to be on the cover of *Vegan Health & Fitness Magazine* for the second time, in January 2013, I was far from prepared for the photo shoot. I had taken six months off from weight training and didn't resemble a bodybuilder in any way. I was told that it didn't matter, that the magazine is about health and fitness, not bodybuilding, but my association with the fitness industry has always been represented as a bodybuilder. I was nervous and unsure how this would go, as I wasn't even comfortable in my own skin at that time. In addition to being absent from the gym for more than six months, I had casually taken up running, and was still reeling from back and wrist injuries that sidelined me in the first place. Furthermore, I had just experienced months of some level of depression as a result of not feeling like myself because of my injuries and muscle loss. On top of that, I hadn't shaved, wasn't tanned, and was surrounded by my peers at a *Vegan Health & Fitness Magazine* Expo where the photo shoot was taking place on the main stage in a conference room for all to see.

My friend Mindy Collette, featured throughout this book, was slated to be on the magazine cover with me and she flew to Los Angeles from Oregon to join me for this appearance. She was in shape as she always is, and was prepared for the photo shoot and we moved forward with it. My partner, Karen, captured some photos while she watched Mindy and me go through the poses for our cover shoot up on the stage. As soon as I saw the photos I confirmed what I already knew, that they were not adequate for the magazine cover. Mindy looked great, but I did not represent myself the way I wanted. Many champion, well-known, and successful plant-based athletes were at the fitness expo, and as an early pioneer in this lifestyle, I felt like I let the community down by being out of shape and a fragile version of my former championship self. Either I was retired for good and it didn't matter anymore that I wasn't in bodybuilding shape, or I could do something about it to show I still had some drive left in me after all these years.

With the exciting opportunity to be the first ever two-time cover model for *Vegan Health & Fitness Magazine*, alongside one of my best friends, I challenged myself to follow the advice I often wrote about in that very magazine and become consistent again.

The day after the unsuccessful photo shoot, I asked the editor of the magazine if we could reshoot the photos two to three months later, and professed a claim of confidence that I could get back into good shape within a 12-week period. When editor, Brenda Carey, confirmed we could do the reshoot for the cover in the spring, I got to work in the gym and in the kitchen. I knew what I was capable of achieving if I followed my own advice of consistent training. After a six to eight month break from the gym, I was ready to start lifting again. I got right down to business the next day and noticed changes taking place quickly. Between the initial photo shoot in late January to the new one in early April, I got ready. I basically treated this period as bodybuilding pre-competition mode. In the morning I performed fat-burning cardiovascular training on an empty stomach four days per week in the form of riding a stationary bike for 25-45 minutes. I lifted weights in the evening five days per week. A few days a week I even did an additional cardiovascular, fat-burning workout after my weight training session, using the stair-stepper for 20-25 minutes. During this period I did not restrict my diet, but I ate the whole foods I enjoyed most, namely, a lot of potatoes, yams, lentils, beans, brown rice, quinoa, leafy greens, and fruit. Nothing about my diet suggested any forms of deprivation that is commonplace in most bodybuilding nutrition programs. I did not restrict carbohydrates, cut water, or follow other traditional bodybuilding competition preparation methods surrounding restriction or deprivation. I simply found an objective to work toward, incorporated my favorite exercises and foods into my lifestyle, and worked hard, knowing there was an end result I was striving for. And if it worked, I knew it could have a positive impact on thousands of people. With my sights set on a far more productive photo shoot for a magazine cover that would be in hundreds or even thousands of stores around the world, I owned up to responsibility, accountability, transparency, and literally put my money where my mouth was and I personally flew Mindy back out to L.A. where I was living at the time, for a reshoot at the magazine's headquarters (before recently moving their office to Austin, TX). I added significant muscle and definition and my confidence in my own physique had returned, all in a matter of weeks. In essence, my whole-food, plant-based meal plan combined with consistent and purpose-driven resistance weight training, and deliberately applied cardiovascular exercise, created a measurable result and positive return on investment. Ultimately, I became happier. Not just because I had a more desirable physical appearance as far as my personal goals were concerned, but because I rediscovered enjoyable exercise designed to achieve a meaningful outcome. And it worked. Exercising regularly helped me overcome the depression, sadness, and frustration I had experienced during my time away from exercise, and naturally, seeing forward progress unfold in front of me was inspiring.

When I flew Mindy back to L.A. for the shoot in April, we both looked like outstanding representatives of the plant-based athlete lifestyle and we had a rewarding photo shoot, knowing our physiques would likely inspire many. Ultimately, the photos from that photo shoot in April did not end up on the cover, but not because we weren't in shape. The lighting turned out to be less than ideal, but luckily we scheduled additional photo shoots during our time in L.A. and some of those photos turned out to be quite popular and have ended up in full-page magazine ads in hundreds of thousands of individual issues. Mindy and I did yet another photo shoot together in Texas in July for a third attempt to get adequate photos for the cover, and indeed we did. Perhaps more of a testament to persistence than anything, we finally made it work. It was rather fitting to have us on the cover together because Mindy and I met at a bodybuilding competition we both competed in back in 2009 and I introduced her to the vegan lifestyle. We quickly became friends and over time she emerged as one of my best friends. Sharing the cover with Mindy and watching her career blossom was perhaps the most rewarding result of this three-month effort to get back in shape. Below are the before and after photos from L.A. from January and April, and the eventual magazine cover. In this case, rather than giving up, the third time was a charm for us and we were on the cover of what turned out to be the bestselling issue of *Vegan Health & Fitness Magazine* of all time.

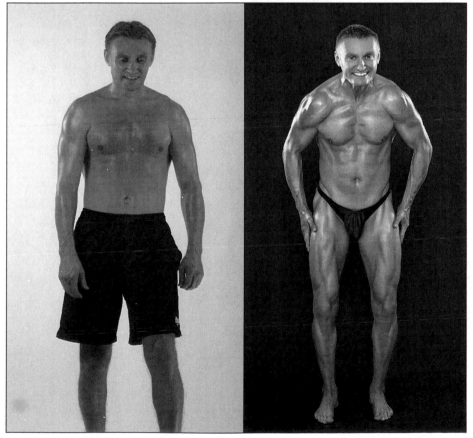

Robert Cheeke - January 2013 Vegan Health & Fitness Magazine photo shoot

Robert Cheeke - April 2013
Photo by Melissa Schwartz
theveganrevolution.net

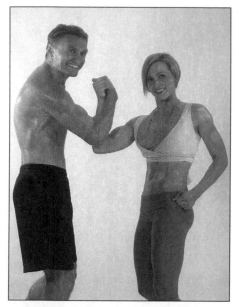

Robert Cheeke and Mindy Collette -
January 2013 *Vegan Health & Fitness*
Magazine photo shoot

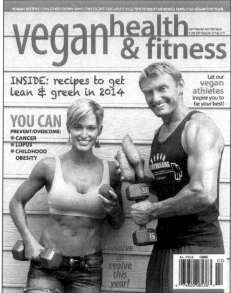

Robert Cheeke and Mindy Collette -
July 2013 photo shoot
Vegan Health & Fitness Magazine cover
Photo by Brenda Carey

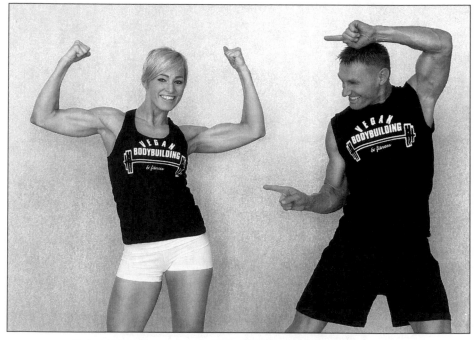

Robert Cheeke and Mindy Collette - April 2013 photo shoot
Photo by Melissa Schwartz - theveganrevolution.net

My transformation over a short period of time helped me achieve something important for me and for my friend, and enhanced both of our careers because we were willing to set specific goals, create action plans with timelines, and work hard to achieve them. I followed the fat-burning and muscle-building formulas discussed in chapters four and five and told my own story through my transformation. It also built my confidence back up. That specific physique transformation was completed in less than 12 weeks and propelled another year of continuous fitness that remains today. I continue to avoid exercises that jeopardize the health of my lower back and wear a protective wrist brace with every workout, but I still manage to train hard and train consistently. I don't let perceived limitations dictate what I can or cannot accomplish as an athlete. Sometimes I have to be creative to find another way to reach a destination, but I put in the time to search for answers and learn from experiences. There are plenty of other transformation stories, far more inspirational than my quest to end up on another magazine cover. The following transformation stories are truly life changing in some incredibly powerful and deeply meaningful ways.

I am proud to share these inspirational transformation stories from my colleagues in the plant-based athlete community. I interviewed the following individuals specifically for this book. This is a summary of who they are and what they have accomplished in their physical transformations. I hope they leave you motivated and inspired to start your own powerful journey to achieve outstanding results in health and fitness.

Transformation #1

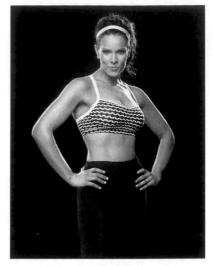

Tricia Kelly

Teacher turned Trainer
From nearly 300 pounds
to fitness model

Tricia Kelly
Photo by Melissa Schwartz
theveganrevolution.net

Although change is often scary, sometimes it can be far more painful to remain the same. If you had asked me a few short years ago where I would be today, my response would have included marriage, a master's degree, and a white picket fence. The reality that I am creating for myself now is very different than what I ever would have anticipated and I could not be happier.

Like many others, I have struggled with food throughout my life. I was never the picture of health; normally eating sweets for breakfast on the way to school. In middle and high school, a typical lunch consisted of two bags of chips, ice cream, and something fried. Food was not something that I thought about. I ate what I liked and what everyone else was eating.

As a young adult, health and wellness were not priorities for me. I was always a strong, tall girl, but not thin like my friends. I was an athlete and a tomboy, so my daily level of activity and participation in competitive athletics kept me in decent shape.

Life and my appearance changed drastically upon my move to Boston and enrollment at the Berklee College of Music. As a result of my unchanged eating habits and a very sedentary lifestyle, my overall health and quality of life deteriorated. My friends and I elected to party; drinking too much alcohol and ordering take out in the early hours of the morning.

During my sophomore year of college, I lost about 50 pounds by adopting a fad low-carbohydrate diet. As many others have experienced, it is very difficult to maintain weight loss by restricting certain food groups completely.

To avoid gaining the weight back but still hoping to indulge in all things I had deprived myself of, I turned to binging and purging. Obviously, this was extremely unhealthy and ineffective. I tried to find a permanent solution through a quick-fix diet, as opposed to an overall lifestyle change.

If only I had turned in my poor habits along with my cap and gown in 2007. By 2010, I weighed over 270 pounds. Following some major life events, including a move across the country, beginning a new job, and finally walking away from a struggling relationship, I had finally had enough. I no longer liked the person I saw when I looked in the mirror.

I became unrecognizable to myself. I was hiding inside baggy, layered clothing. I was tired of being held back by other people, other things, and most of all my weight. I wanted to find myself again and get on the right track to go after my dreams and live the life I have always imagined.

In the summer of 2011, I made my health a priority. I began attending boot camp fitness classes with some of my friends. After getting back into a fitness routine, I was ready to tackle my eating. I made changes slowly, adopting a vegetarian diet, and eating a lot of greens. I was on a path to achieving optimal health and wanted to do everything possible to live my best life.

By March 2012, boot camp instructor, and friend, Chad Byers suggested that I read *The China Study* and watch several documentaries including *Forks Over Knives*. After doing my own reading and speaking with Chad about it, my mind was made up. Extensive research has proven that many degenerative diseases can be controlled and in some cases, even reversed, by adopting a whole-food, plant-based diet. I could only wonder: if diet would reverse disease, what could it do for a seemingly healthy person?

I was determined to find out and have not looked back. Since making one of the best decisions of my life and becoming vegan, I have become stronger and leaner than ever before. I know I am doing the best thing for my body —not to mention environmental and ethical issues. I have compassion for animals and am now an advocate for vegan and cruelty-free living in all areas. It is 100 percent possible to live a full, healthy, and strong life without harming other living things. There is no need to take beautiful things from the world in order to improve ourselves.

In July 2012, I began taking my physical transformation even more seriously and started training every day, alternating between strength training days and High Intensity Interval Training (HIIT) conditioning days. I follow a split routine consisting of three workouts: 1) Legs, 2) Back and Biceps, and 3) Chest, Shoulders and Triceps. I eat a high raw diet consisting mainly of dark leafy greens, fresh green vegetable juices, fruit smoothies, and whole plant foods.

Molding, shaping, and recreating my physical body was a priority for a few years, but I realized that there was a lot more I needed to do to live my best life. I dedicated a bit of time to do some soul searching to find my purpose and live with intention. Initially, I moved to Austin, TX to work as a teacher. I became a music teacher because it came easily to me. Education and music were two of my passions, so it seemed like a logical career choice.

Natural. Easy. Logical. These are not the words that move me. In fact, they do nothing for me. These words do not speak to me and certainly do not rattle me to the core. After four years as an Elementary Music Specialist in Austin, I realized I was settling. I was playing it safe.

Since beginning this amazing journey a few years ago, I have done every possible thing to improve my life and become the best version of myself. Within this past two years, I fell so deeply in love with health and fitness that I began coaching part time at a gym opened by Chad Byers, called Beyond Fit. I wanted to be there all the time. Motivating others to reach their goals and pushing them to do things they never thought they could do before resonated so deeply with me and in a way nothing else has. Transitioning to coaching full time was always a part of the plan, but I did not know when would be the right time.

I spent some time in reflection and thought about when the best time would be. How could I stay in a teaching job that no longer fed my soul or touched my heart? How could I live my best life when I was so unhappy with how I was spending my days? How could I be an effective coach if I was not brave enough to go after all that I wanted? I could not continue on that path. I refused to do so. I held the power and decided that there was no time like the present. I punched fear in the face and resigned from teaching in May 2013.

Beyond Fit is my favorite place in the world. Each and every day I wake up and look forward to working with the community I have built with the owner and other vegan coach, Chad Byers. We are a dream team; training, coaching, and spreading the plant-based message. We lead by example and want to help others learn that you can build a powerhouse physique and live as healthy as possible without harming animals or the environment. Do not hold back. I urge you to begin living your best life now. It is a beautiful process; developing and unfolding a little bit at a time. There is no better time than the present to decide exactly who you want to be and begin living it.

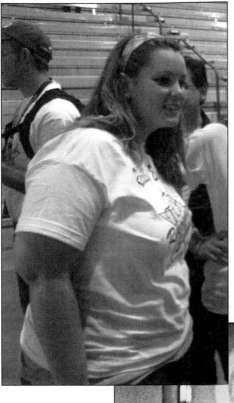

Tricia Kelly - 2009

Tricia Kelly - 2014

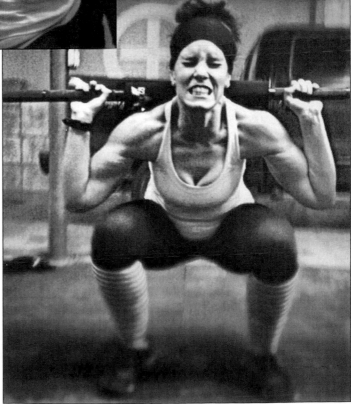

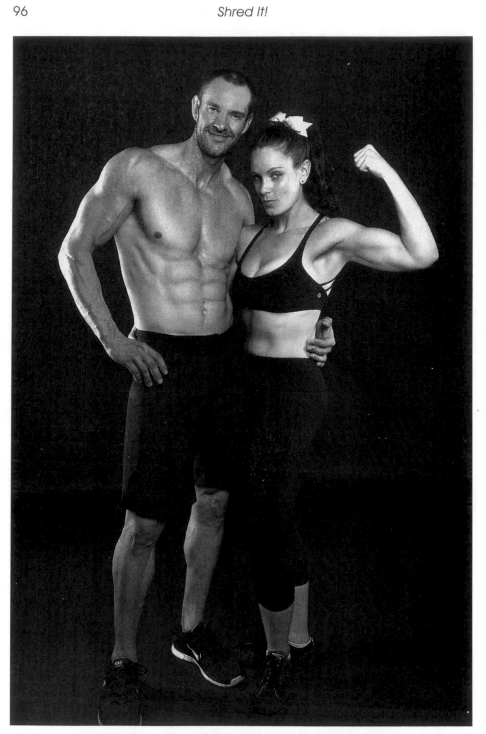

Tricia Kelly and Chad Byers - Photo by Anna MG Photography

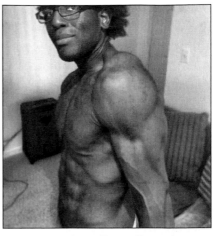

Larry Bennett

Transformation #2

Larry Bennett

From 300+ pounds to ripped 175-pound health coach

I began to gain weight in fourth grade and was obese by the time I entered sixth grade, partly because I spent the early part of my life extremely sedentary. I spent hours staring at the television while enjoying the action and adventure of several much-loved video games. I can remember days when I'd literally fall asleep with the controller in my hands, then wake up an hour later only to resume my gaming marathon. When you combine this kind of behavior with unhealthy eating habits, weight gain is inevitable. My family and I honestly had no clue about nutrition back then. A burger was a burger, fries were fries, and cookies were cookies. That is how we ate. The problem is, nutrition isn't really taught in our public education system, so in what way were we supposed to know to what extent hydrogenated trans fats, enriched and refined carbohydrates, Recombinant Bovine Growth Hormone (rbGH), Insulin-like Growth Factor-1 (IGF-1), Monosodium Glutamate (MSG), and how hundreds of other artificial additives, preservatives, and pesticides can wreak havoc on the human body? Unfortunately, because of our lack of knowledge, we suffered greatly.

People tend to ask me all the time, "What made you want to change?" or "Why did you decide to do it?" Well, it all came down to one mind-shifting incident. While I was sitting beside my brother, Micah, in my parents' room watching television, something extremely hilarious came on screen that caused me to laugh hysterically. I suddenly regained consciousness while face first on the floor. After regaining my awareness, I cleaned up the bowl of chili and white rice I had been eating for dinner and asked Micah what happened. My first thought was that I had somehow fallen asleep, but Micah said, "When you passed out, your eyes were wide open."

After that incident, I began to worry constantly because I felt like a walking time bomb. I used to think that my day of reckoning might just be around the corner. At some point, there came a time when I started to lose interest in life. My emotions had numbed and I didn't see any reason to continue living. I was dealing with high blood pressure, heartburn, arthritis, and constipation with blood in the stool, unnatural allergies with bags full of tissues to combat it, joint pain and cramps, deep snoring, bad breath, adrenal fatigue, symptoms of bipolar disorder, and low self-esteem.

For the majority of my life, I walked on the passage of obesity. I exhausted every attempt I had to lose weight, and eventually lost control of who I was. One night, while feeling lonely, depressed, and miserable, I began to interrogate God, "Why me? Why is this happening to me?" I tried to hold back my wreck of emotions, but something else was in command of me that night, "How come I am so fat? Why can't I be normal?" With tears covering my face, I brought forth every ounce of willpower I could gather, and basically suppressed my feelings and accepted my fate. This was not an isolated occurrence, and each time it happened, I'd delve further and further into desolation; entering the lowest point in my life.

The true turning point came when my brother, Timothy, came home from Florida to visit us on my parents' land in Pine Hills, Alabama. After catching up with him, Micah and I decided to go on a short vacation. We drove back to Florida with Timothy and ended up staying, permanently. Shortly afterwards, I was hired by Whole Foods Market in Tampa, as a retail grocery team member. It was an absolute culture shock! This was the first time I had ever been exposed to such a mind-boggling reality. I was finally introduced to the world of healthy eating that unleashed a flow of overwhelming hope.

What's amazing is that around the same time, Timothy was accepted into the Whole Foods Market: Total Health Immersion Program in Santa Rosa, California. Before he went to spend six days with Dr. John McDougall and his wife, Mary McDougall, authors of *The Starch Solution*, we both made a promise to go on this exotic vegan diet together. On the day before Timothy's return, I went on a fast food eating spree! I binged on burgers, fries, soda, pizza, fried rice, chicken, and big beef burritos all day. That same night, I remembered how active I used to be in my first few years of school, before I started to put on weight. I could run laps around the schoolyard effortlessly and never ran out of what seemed like immeasurable energy. That was probably the most active time of my life. Reflecting back on that much healthier time, I knew I needed to change my lifestyle to achieve the life I wanted. I didn't want to feel sick anymore, I wanted to feel alive again, like those early days on the playground. The want and need to have that back in my life is what stopped the paradox. Thus, a new man was born.

I spent the next couple months in total commitment to my new vegan lifestyle: I refused samples of processed food that were offered to me from coworkers; I cooked 80 percent of my meals from home and ate the other 20 percent from the Whole Foods salad bar; I eliminated the use of salt, sugar, and oil; and I allowed my passion, the obligation to better myself, to fuel me throughout the journey. What's truly important is that I was never afraid of not being able to ever eat the junk I used to. In fact, I wrote them off as my enemies, while actual whole foods grew to be my allies. Over time, my taste buds adapted. I began to crave whole grains, legumes, fruits, nuts, seeds, and leafy greens. I tell people all the time that my discipline was probably equal to that of a Buddhist monk, possibly more. Within six months, I changed my life forever, shedding 135 pounds of fat from my body indefinitely. Fast forward to today, and I'm liberated from a total of 150 pounds of fat. I've literally lost the equivalence of a whole person from my body! You too, can make a change in your life. Have you ever asked yourself, "Why should I accept what is not wanted?"

Now as an avid member of the Vegan Bodybuilding & Fitness community, I seek to prove that you can build muscle and be extremely fit on a whole-food, plant-based diet. My methods of training arc based on gymnastics and bodyweight strength. As for meals, I keep them fairly simple. Here's the basic meal plan I use on a daily basis:

Breakfast:
Steel-cut oats, chopped apricots, and an 8-ounce banana date smoothie

Lunch:
Brown rice, lentils, and hummus wrapped in steamed collard leaves

Dinner:
Coconut water-sautéed broccoli, kale, quinoa with an 8-ounce bean smoothie

Snacks:
2 tbsp of almond butter, 5-10 Medjool dates, and a live probiotic

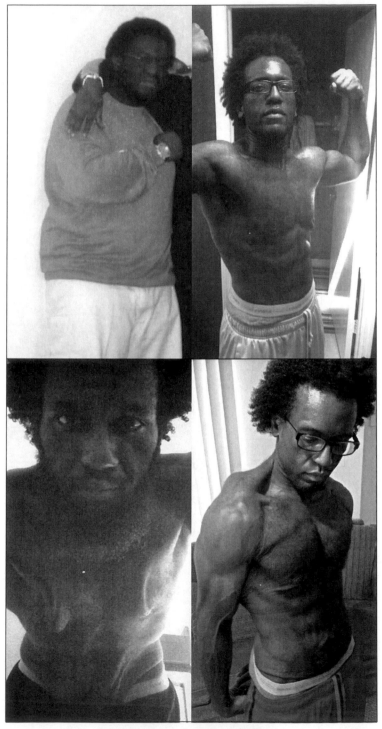

Larry Bennett - Before and after

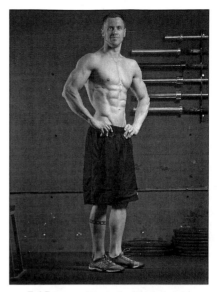

Transformation #3

Ed Bauer

Becoming Someone with Something to Prove

Ed Bauer - Photo by Mark Rainha

Can I be honest? I am a little hesitant to puts words on this document because I am not a writer. At least that's what I've told myself. I have told myself a lot of things. In fact, what I really have said to myself my whole life is, I am average. I am not good at anything. I am not too bad at anything. I am not that smart. I am not that fast. I am not that funny. I am not that anything. I am just plain, nothing more, nothing less. This is what the voice in my head was telling me. This is no fault of my parents. Both of them raised me and supported me in whatever I wanted to do. My father always said I could be anything I wanted to be.

Be that as it may, the society I grew up in told me a different story. It told me that very few people succeed in life, some people fail miserably, but most fall in the middle. Most never make as much money as they want, are not as effective as they want, or as happy as they could be. This seemed like a very likely reality for me. My mind left me somewhere in the middle, just trying to keep my head above water.

I got into hardcore music when I was fifteen years old through some of my skateboarding friends. I was then introduced to the straight-edge lifestyle (a lifetime commitment to be drug and alcohol free) and eventually veganism. Hardcore music usually took on a radically political stance, so these ideas were fairly well-expressed in the mid-'90s. I first became straight-edge to take better care of myself. I later became vegan because I wanted to take better care of the world around me. From this existence, I had the urge to spread the message of compassionate veganism. I didn't feel effective holding banners and protesting. It didn't seem to speak to my passion. Instead of shaming people or scaring them in a negative manner, I knew I wanted to lead by a positive example. I later realized that fitness was the answer.

After graduating college with a four-year degree, from age twenty-two to about twenty-five, my life was sort of passing me by. I didn't know who I was or who I wanted to be. Really, this lack of purpose was a lack of confidence, disguised as normal life. I didn't yet realize it, but it was really up to me to decide what life I was going to live. It wasn't society and its perceived limitations; I was numb and essentially paralyzed by my own thoughts. Once I realized what was happening to me, I started to branch out and push myself more. I started taking more chances. I decided that I wanted to be a change in this world. As a compassionate vegan, I wanted to inspire people to take a look at what they were eating and how they were affecting the world around them. I wanted people to see that a vegan lifestyle can make you healthy, strong, more attractive, and more confident. Fitness became my tool to share the compassionate vegan message with the world around me.

Our habits make us who we are tomorrow. For me, I still have ingrained in me some of my eating habits from when I was an unhealthy teenager. I grew up around big guys who knew how to eat…a lot. My brother, my dad, and my best friend all weighed 240 pounds or more and were at least six feet tall. I was 165 pounds and five feet nine, trying to keep up with these guys. That led to the wrong habits for sure. I still like a lot of the foods I ate back then. I still like sugary cereal, sandwiches, fried food, candy, and cookies, but now I know how that stuff affects me. Some people think that I have always been fit or always looked a certain way. I want to let you know the real story. I have never been that overweight, but I surely wasn't fit. It wasn't until 2009 that I truly pushed myself to see who I could be. If you never try, then it is guaranteed. You will never know who you can be, or what you can achieve. I am reminded of Henry Ford's quote, "Whether you think you can, or you think you can't—you're right."

Back then (2009), I had just moved to Portland, OR and got a job as a personal trainer at 24 Hour Fitness. I knew I wanted to get in the best shape of my life, and started my journey. Along the way, I met Robert Cheeke, and he challenged me to see what I can do on a bodybuilding stage. Not yet confident enough to step on the stage, I decided to replicate the experience, without the stage. I got my close friend Randall Perez to agree to be my photographer for a photo shoot. We set the date and it was on. It was within this context of mental focus and determination that I was able to make the initial transformation from being a regular looking guy, to an example of what a strong vegan diet and training regimen can accomplish. After the photo shoot, with encouragement from friends including Robert, I took this confidence and entered in a bodybuilding competition in May 2010. That focus and determination earned me 1st Place in the Novice Middleweight Bodybuilding category. I went from an existence of feeling forgettable, average, uninspired, and questionably satisfied with anything, to knowing that I truly can succeed if I put my mind to it. Since getting shredded that first time in 2009, with the tremendous support of Robert and www.vegan-bodybuilding.com, I have managed to stay one of the leading faces and (still working on) voices in the vegan fitness movement.

Every day, I decide if I want to push myself to become something better, or let old habits turn me back into who I once was. Every day, with persistence, I decide if I am going to exercise and do it with purpose. I decide if I am going to eat cleanly focus on quality nutrients. Every day, I have to decide if I will sleep enough and recover properly. I decide whether I continue to educate myself on proper fitness and nutrition. With understanding of how this process works, I decide that pain is temporary and necessary for anything worth accomplishing. I think of the Robert Allen quote, "Everything you want is just outside your comfort zone." Old habits die hard, and I know that. It never gets easy, but we decide who we can be, every day. Embrace the challenge, and let it redefine you. I am happy to get the chance to promote a compassionate world through fitness and awareness. I hope you will join me and do the same.

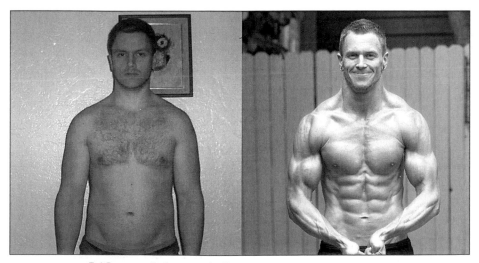

Ed Bauer - Before and after - After photo by Randall Perez

Transformation #4

Elana Priesman

Lost the pregnancy weight plus a whole lot more!

Elana's "Plantsformation"

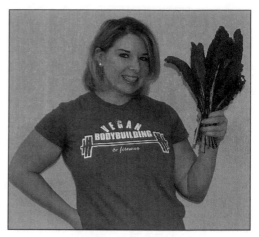

Elana Priesman

I struggled with weight and health issues my entire life. I believe fate brought me to meet accomplished plant-based athletes, Rip Esselstyn, Robert Cheeke, and Chad Byers all on the same night. After watching documentaries like *Forks Over Knives* and *Fat, Sick and Nearly Dead*, I had tried to discuss the plant-based diet with doctors and nutritionists and they did not support it. I actually had a doctor try to convince me to go on a Paleo diet, a current fad diet tied in to the CrossFit lifestyle. Luckily, I met these three men the very next week, which was August 30, 2012, and my life was forever changed. I had never been exposed to fit men before who didn't eat meat. I was astounded! I have since lost over 80 pounds, and will soon be celebrating my 100-pound total weight loss. After seven years of my cholesterol being in the 260s to 280s, it plummeted to below 200. My diabetes and insulin resistance disappeared, too. Not only that, but I feel incredible every day, have a ton of energy, and work out eight times a week.

My passion is to educate others about the amazing aspects of plant-based nutrition! I feel empowered and enlightened. I love giving my body what it needs with plant strong nutrition. I feel so much more alive not putting dead energy from dead animals in my body. I also obtained my certification in Plant-Based Nutrition from the T. Colin Campbell Foundation at Cornell University.

In addition, I am beyond thrilled to have been exposed to this whole new world of people. Every day my life has renewed meaning and purpose to push myself harder and educate myself more and more. My goal is to be the change that I wish to see in the world, and to use my body as an example that this *is* possible! I am still on my journey and wish to lose another 15-20 pounds and get more defined. I aim to help inspire others by leading with a positive example. I know I can accomplish that.

It wasn't easy, but it had to be done. I was sick and I was tired; tired of being fat and tired of being unhealthy. I had to be accountable to myself, and I had to be around for my young daughter. I needed to make a serious change, and I did. After hearing Robert Cheeke and Chad Byers speak at an Engine 2 Potluck dinner in Austin, TX on that August evening, it all made sense. Meat and dairy had no place in my life. Eliminating them completely from my diet was something I had never thought of, something I had never even tried fully. I had attempted dabbling with vegan meals here and there, but had never completely abstained from those foods with a lifetime commitment.

I was so excited to change my health and body that I rushed home and stayed up watching a video on how to make bean burgers produced by renowned plant-based nutritionist Jeff Novick. I didn't know anything about the new path I was about to embark on, because once I became accountable to myself, I knew nothing else mattered, and I ate those same bean burgers the entire week: for breakfast, lunch, and dinner until I had the time to figure out my next plant-based recipe.

Within days I was at the Beyond Fit training facility with my new buff and handsome trainer, Chad Byers. You know you are out of shape when you can barely survive the warm up. I remember coming home after my first class, fainting onto the couch and lying there for an hour. I was exhausted!

I feel like I have come a long way since then, and I now crave those workouts, and do double sessions often. I can remember what it felt like to use just the bar as my working weight, and now I am adding more plates than my own body weight in some exercises.

I have measured my success through getting Dexa scans and keeping track of my body measurements and using an Omron handheld body fat measuring device. The Dexa scans give me an overall view of my muscle mass and more insight than the external measurements. I also wore a BodyMedia device for a long time to get an idea of how many calories I was burning during a typical day. Even though I have not tracked my meals every single day, I eat the same meals over and over, so it just becomes second nature, knowing what I am consuming to make sure I am getting my desired macronutrients met through nutrition in order to achieve my goals. I have experimented with several types of plant-based diets. I started out with an Engine 2 style (a low fat, vegan nutrition plan that cuts out vegetable oils – a diet created by former professional triathlete and firefighter, Rip Esselstyn). I then shifted to removing all forms of gluten and starchy carbohydrates to see how my body would respond, and I delved into 80/10/10 raw fruitarian diet for a short term too. I learned a lot about my body and how it responds to various meals.

They say everyone is different, and I am still getting to know myself, and as I change, my needs are also constantly changing. I pay attention to nutrient timing, and it takes of lot of discipline to always plan ahead. The biggest part of my success is attributed to my willpower of being responsible for my own meals. Like a baby who needs a diaper bag, I need my food bag. I travel a lot and have to bring my blender and a suitcase of food with me. I have had to tell people I have food allergies sometimes, just to make things easier. I have had TSA agents search me just so I could bring hummus aboard a plane. I rarely go to restaurants, and even when I do, I will order just steamed vegetables or a custom salad. I bring my own food with me 98 percent of the time wherever I go. I'm not going to say it's easy, it does take effort, but I'm not going to let social events and excuses get in my way. I have enjoyed some food off my diet a few times during the year too. I attended two Engine 2 Diet health conferences where the food was entirely plant-based, but a little more calorie dense than I typically enjoy. At those events, I understand they are trying to appeal to people who are new to the lifestyle and they cater the events with the best recipes in their arsenal.

I also stay on top of getting my blood work checked. I like to ensure I am keeping up to date with my hormones to see that my levels are improving. I have had some roadblocks with my thyroid, and I believe getting it in balance is an essential part of this health process.

A typical day for me looks like this: I intermittent fast until about 12:30 pm, and my first meal is green juice (usually), and a big power greens salad with nutritional yeast and salsa with cilantro on top, or a pre-washed salad blend of arugula and spinach with fresh strawberries and blueberries on top with hemp seeds and a few walnuts. I recently discovered this amazing oil- and fat-free salad dressing by Braggs that I enjoy. I also have made my own salad dressings out of blended fruits and vegetables. Occasionally I will add avocado too, but not always. My second meal is the same, or a vegetable with the same toppings. My other meals are just fruit and vegetables. I feel my best when I am eating raw due to the convenience of being able to grab and go. I feel like my body is getting a straight shot of nutrients that makes me feel energetic and not too bogged down by digestion so I can get my workout on.

I get contacted often from people struggling with staying focused on their diets. People get very upset with themselves when they feel their eating is out of control. A lot of people think I have some sort of super powers when it comes to being so disciplined. It is one thing to be vegan, and it is a whole different thing to be a whole-food, plant-based vegan. It is really easy to eat junk food, and there are, in fact, teams of scientists that design food to be addictive with the fat, sugar, and salt trifecta. Those foods may be fun to eat once in a while, but in reality if you want to perform well in the gym, and feel your ultimate best self, there is not much room to indulge, because in my personal experience, the more you eat of those filler foods, the less you have room for the nutrient dense foods your body requires to perform at its best. This is something you will just know when you experience it. I advise people to do their own experiments to see how they feel. Another important part of the equation is staying hydrated with a lot of water. It will aid in regulating cravings and just make you feel incredible. I aim to drink a gallon a day of pure water. One last piece of advice is to create a vision board and put photos of fruits and vegetables on it. You can look at it daily, and even think of it as a menu of your choices. The more you look at the visual images, the more conscious you become. You make it your choice. You have the power, and can master your destiny of how you want to fuel your body.

I am sometimes shocked at the person I have become. I used to question my purpose in life. Being able to inspire others and help others transform their lives from following my example gives so much meaning to my life. Now I feel empowered, I feel important, I feel like I am making a difference in the world. I feel like the luckiest person to have the right people in my corner. My greatest joy will be when someday someone tells me they were able to save their life because of me. It is all a circle; we can save people, the people save animals, and so on. I am grateful for the opportunity to meet all the people mentioned above who have lived their truths, so I could be able to just live. I really believe it was meant for me. I love this life.

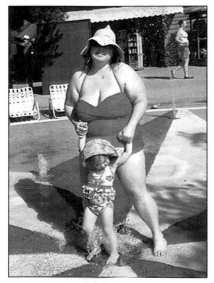

Elana Priesman
Before a plant-based diet

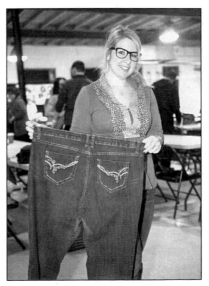

Elana Priesman
After a plant-based diet

Transformation #5

Aaron MacNeil

From out of shape father to Super Dad!

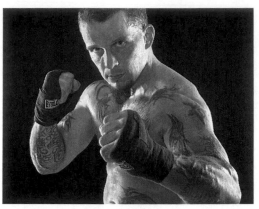

Aaron MacNeil
Photo by Victoria Prince

I would like to start off about four years ago when I first started to think about my health, and my family's health, and what direction I wanted to take. I was your ordinary guy who worked 7:00 am to 5:00 pm, came home, had a few beers, maybe some BBQ food, watched some television, and called it a night. I started to notice that I was slowly getting heavier and not really doing much physical activity outside of work at all. It was the same old excuse that I never really had any time for anything else in my life. My breathing problems just kept getting worse and I was even booked for surgery for my sinus cavities, as they were completely closed over and I was having a really hard time breathing. I started researching and looking into solutions, studying food, and the effects it has on the body. This changed my family's lives.

The first thing I did to improve my health was cut out dairy from my diet and this is when things started to become clear to me. I did this for four weeks and was very surprised that my sinus symptoms were gone. My sinuses cleared up, and for the first time in years, I could breathe normally through my nose. I found the same results with my two daughters. They had asthma, or dairy-induced lung inflammation, as we now call it. My younger daughter had asthma bad enough to take puffers a few times a day during the colder weather and suffered at least one chest infection every winter. After about six weeks, we noticed my younger daughter not reaching for her puffer as much, and after a couple more weeks she didn't need it at all, and hasn't used it in three and a half years, and has not suffered one chest infection. Aside from sports-related injuries, my daughters haven't been to the doctor in just as long. This is all because of food choices our family made. Amazing!

I started exercising and taking care of myself, and taking one week at a time to try to feel better and get healthy. The good thing about this was that

I had my family's support because we all switched to a plant-based diet at the same time. They didn't have much of a choice, considering that I am the cook. My body was getting stronger, I was able to do things I could never do before, I was lifting more weight in the gym, and I was feeling better than I had in years. It seemed like my energy levels went from incredibly low to off the charts. I pushed hard for about six months until I was just programmed to do these healthy activities every day.

Fueling my body with clean, nutrient-dense plants made it easy for me to have these crazy workouts and then work a labor-intensive ten-hour workday, and my recovery was amazing. I was making gains that I would never have thought were possible, given my previous health conditions. When your body has all the resources it needs to grow and repair, it just becomes so much easier to progress and make gains. I can run for kilometers like it's a walk in the park, and I could never do that before. I couldn't walk up the stairs without getting winded. I weighed 245 pounds before I made the switch, and I dropped down to 160 pounds in the first six months. The fat just melted off. After adopting a weight-training program, I am up to 185 pounds, but my fat percentage is still low.

I do a combination of high intensity weight training with heavy weights, and with light weights, changing my approach every other week. I am a big fan of interval training. This really works for me to always keep me in a fat-burning state. I usually do twenty minutes of interval training in the morning and another twenty minutes of interval training in the evening. My workout is usually one and a half hours long. My current approach is for the first 40 minutes I usually do a split training routine, which is training back and biceps or chest and triceps with weights. I am always changing it up. I try to train one muscle group while another muscle group can rest during the same workout. For example, I will do a back exercise, then a biceps exercise, and then return to a back exercise, and repeat. I limit my rest in between sets with this approach. So after about the 40-minute range I start to throw in some interval training on every third set I do for another 30 minutes. Then for the last 20 minutes, I like to just hit the interval training hard until I can't do anymore. It can be hard at first but is very rewarding, especially for me.

I am very proud of my three young vegan fitness ambassadors, my kids. My seven-year-old daughter trains 12 hours a week in competitive gymnastics, my nine-year-old daughter plays hockey 3-4 times a week and is currently the top scorer for her team, and my eighteen-year-old son loves working out in the gym at school every day and is passionate about boxing. Seeing my kids thrive is so rewarding and we no longer get the advice from others about how they need meat and dairy to live. My wife, Heather, is the backbone of the family. She is my best friend and without her I would have never achieved any of my goals. From the moment we met my life has changed so much for the better. She is always making sure the kids have fun foods available every day, never missing a day, which is a big bonus because when trying to make fun healthy choices sometimes you get stumped, but she never does. Her work toward raising a healthy family is relentless and she never takes a day off. She is a true role model and hero in our family.

My eating style is very calculated. I always make sure my meals are pre-made and ready to go in my cooler. I find that failure to prepare meals is a common mistake a lot of people tend to make. I always have a cooler with all of my favorite meals packed and ready to go and another one for the kids if we are out together. We don't have any vegan restaurants close to where we live, and we obviously haven't eaten in a fast food place since we switched to a plant-based diet, so preparation is imperative. I find that portion control and eating more meals during the day makes a huge difference as well. It really isn't that complicated once you get the hang of it. I try to eat as many whole foods as I possibly can, minimizing anything that is processed, that has refined sugar or empty calories.

Recently, I have been approached at the gym for advice on working out, which always leads to a discussion about nutrition. There is so much misconception out there about following a plant-based diet, which makes me love sharing my story and workout and nutritional advice so much more. I want to help anyone that wants to feel the best they can.

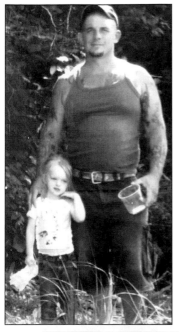

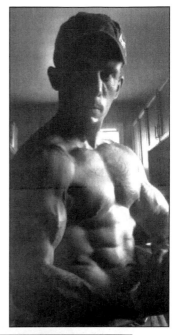

Aaron MacNeil
Before
and
After

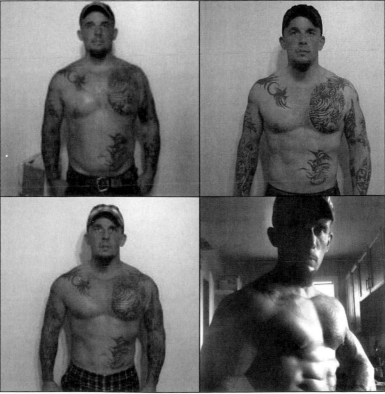

Aaron MacNeil - Transformation collage

Transformation #6

Arvid Beck

Finding a Low Protein Diet for Bodybuilding Success

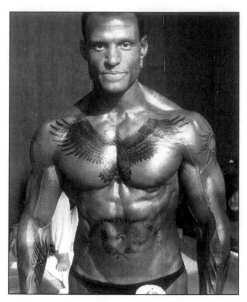

Arvid Beck

Before I decided to take part in my most recent bodybuilding competition, I hadn't been on stage for a while and had put on a lot of weight. I never take any breaks from training, but I had gained a lot of fat during the off-season. I was up to about 98 kilograms (approximately 216 pounds), and I knew I'd have to face a tough diet program to get in shape in time to be adequately prepared for the contest.

I had already taken part in quite a few competitions, so I started my usual carbohydrate-restricted diet, which is the norm in competitive bodybuilding. Although I made some progress, I started to feel sluggish and lightheaded more often, which was nothing new to me, but I got more and more annoyed by these low carbohydrate side effects.

That was the point in which I started to experiment with my diet, by decreasing the amount of protein and fat while increasing my carbohydrate intake. In the beginning, I was a bit skeptical as to whether this could work, but to my surprise, it did. Although I started to eat a lot of carbohydrates, which I never did during former contest diets, and cut out all protein shakes, I constantly lost weight (which was my goal) and had no problems with my recovery. I actually felt better than ever before during a bodybuilding contest preparation.

In the end, everything worked out pretty well. I dropped bodyweight from almost 98 kilograms to 80 kilograms over a period of eighteen weeks, and was able to present myself in really good shape on the bodybuilding stage.

Since then, I never restricted my carbohydrate intake again. Meanwhile, I follow a high carbohydrate, low fat diet year round. I eat lots of whole foods and don't use any protein powders or oils. I also read several books by Dr. John McDougall, Dr. Douglas Graham, Dr. Neal Barnard, Dr. Caldwell Esselstyn, and others, which convinced me that a diet high in carbohydrates, with only little to moderate amounts of protein and fat, is not only good for your athletic performance and physique, but most of all, good for your health.

My typical macronutrient ratio looks like this now:

Carbohydrates	75-80%
Protein	10-15%
Fat	10%

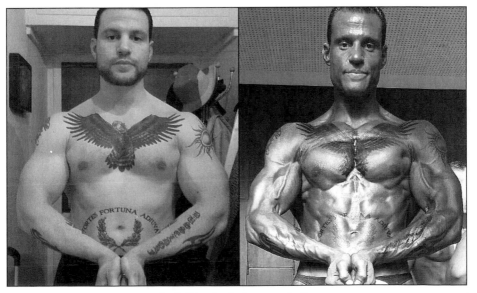

Arvid Beck - Before and after

To read more plant-based athlete transformations, visit the following links, which feature hundreds of inspirational transformation stories:

veganbodybuilding.com/?page=bios

veganbodybuilding.com/forum/viewforum.php?f=48

facebook.com/groups/VeganBodybuildingAndFitness/

We all have the capacity to create our own transformation story in the areas of health and fitness. We can follow the same approach to transform in many areas of life too. How did these transformation stories impact you? What do you aspire to achieve? What story do you want to tell? You can do it. Take action and make it happen!

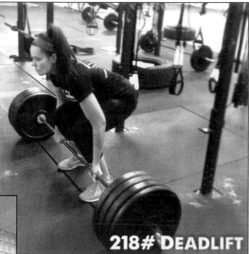

Tricia Kelly -
Deadlifting 218 pounds

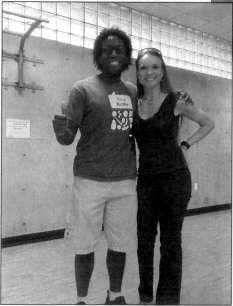

Larry Bennet and Jojo Hulett -
Photo by Robert Cheeke

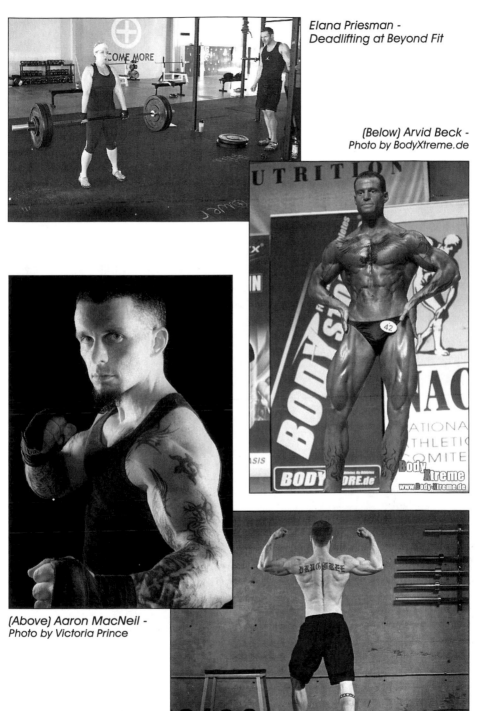

Elana Priesman - Deadlifting at Beyond Fit

(Below) Arvid Beck - Photo by BodyXtreme.de

(Above) Aaron MacNeil - Photo by Victoria Prince

Ed Bauer Photo by Mark Rainha

– CHAPTER 8 –

Whole-Food Meal Plans to get Shredded

> *"There are no nutrients in animal-based foods that are not better obtained from plant-based foods."*
>
> — Dr. T. Colin Campbell, Foremost Nutrition Scientist and bestselling Author of *The China Study*

I used to consume some pretty ridiculous high-calorie meals. I basically put peanut butter on everything early in my bodybuilding career, to the point where I don't really even like peanut butter now, and never buy it. I also ate soy-everything I could find. I celebrated the fact that in one day I consumed eighteen tofu hot dogs. Try to beat that! I pounded a lot of protein drinks back then too, even though I have a small bladder.

Today I cringe when I flip through my first book, *Vegan Bodybuilding & Fitness,* and see meal plans exceeding 6,000 daily calories, which often included lots of supplements and processed foods. Though that high calorie approach worked for me, and has worked for many readers of that book, looking back, I would do things a lot differently now. Enter this chapter, starting anew.

I think it is important to recognize when we learn, grow, and adapt over time. Through various experiences I have been humbled, realizing I didn't know nearly as much as I thought I did, and I have taken my pursuit of knowledge more seriously than I did when I first got involved in body-building and when I first started writing. I credit Dr. T. Colin Campbell, Dr. Caldwell Esselstyn, Brian Wendel, and the Forks Over Knives community for encouraging me, enlightening me, and for teaching me a lot about healthy plant-based nutrition. Registered dietitian George Eisman and Dr. Michael Greger have been additional role models I have shared the speaking stage with numerous times. Their leadership helped me grow and improve my own approach to health and fitness. I have taken the inspirational, scientifically supported information I learned from my role models, and have applied it in my own life to benefit my athletic performance and overall health.

The General Rules to Follow

A general rule to follow is to consume six meals a day, eating every three hours or so. This will keep your body constantly nourished and will help you avoid under eating, overeating, and help you maintain a productive metabolism. It will also ensure you are fueled to workout essentially anytime. Plan this into your meal preparations so you have meals prepared in advance and have access to high levels of nutrition any time of day, regardless of where you are. Keeping whole fruits and vegetables and nut and seed bars with you is an effective way to have healthy fast food while living a busy life on the go. I rarely go anywhere without packing snacks to take with me, consisting of bananas, apples, oranges, berries and other whole foods.

If you consume adequate caloric quantities based on your Basal Metabolic Rate (BMR), you should be able to put on mass, increase muscle, and build strength. You can also get shredded by knowing the proper nutrition approaches to follow, and by implementing them. A low fat nutrition program will likely keep your body fat low. A high-energy nutrition program will keep your energy high. A diverse and calorically sufficient nutrition program will help you recover from exercise efficiently and build muscle. It really can be that easy.

First you'll need to establish how many calories you are burning per day by using a Harris-Benedict calculator, as discussed in Chapter Five. Based on your age, gender, height, weight, and activity level you will find out how many calories you'll need to consume to maintain weight. Given this data you can figure out how many calories you'll need to consume to lose weight, gain muscle, or stay the same. By doing so, you can construct your meal plans according to your goals, based on real, tangible data designed to support your endeavors in a measurable way.

Some categories of foods to consume based on their nutritional impact include:

Fruits – Great for snacks and pre-workout fuel and for energy in general

Starches (Vegetables, Grains, Legumes) – Great as main courses

Greens – Great for overall nutrition

Vegetables – Great for snacks, for main courses, for overall nutrition and variety

Legumes – Great heavy base for filling meals

Nuts/Seeds – Great source of calories and essential fats, quick easy snack

A helpful tip is to prepare large quantities of specific staple foods to last for multiple days. This will save you time and money in the long run and allow more time for exercising, stretching, working, spending time with family, or whatever activities you prioritize. Some of those foods include:

Brown rice	Yams
Quinoa	Soup
Barley	Chili
Beans	Salad
Lentils	Nut and seed trail mix
Potatoes	Granola

Having some of these prepared staples, plus lots of fresh produce, such as fruits and vegetables, makes it easy to prepare filling meals any time.

Additionally, having accessory foods such as avocado, hummus, olives, mushrooms, spreads, dips, and other foods that often get included into snacks or main courses will help enhance the variety and flavor of meals you prepare. You'll want these items to be oil-free since oil is pure fat at 4,000 calories per pound!

Good Breakfast Options

Fruit	Miso soup with greens
Oats	Steamed greens
Grits	Brown rice
Green smoothie	Breakfast burrito
Fruit smoothie	Breakfast wrap
Potatoes/yams	Yerba mate

Good Snack Options

Fruit	Avocado rolls
Vegetables	Fresh vegetable wraps/soft spring rolls
Nuts/seeds	Edamame
Hummus	Almond butter or other nut butters
Smoothie	Fruit, nut and seed trail mix
Flax crackers	Homemade whole-food bars
Dried fruit	Green salad
Prepared food leftovers	Fruit Salad

Good Lunch Options

Starches (beans, lentils, brown rice, potatoes)

Quinoa

Vegetables

Green salad

Fruits

Soup

Fresh salad rolls

Avocado rolls/plant-based sushi

Hummus wrap

Burrito bowl

International foods including plant-based friendly options from Indian, Thai, Ethiopian, Mexican, Japanese, North African, Vietnamese, and Chinese cuisine

Good Dinner Options

Starches (beans, lentils, brown rice, potatoes)

Quinoa

Vegetables

Green salad

Fruits

Soup

Chili

Stuffed bell peppers

Portobello mushrooms

Plant-based burgers, wraps, burritos, or other whole foods

All-you-can-eat plant-based buffets (Indian, Mediterranean, Chinese)

International foods including plant-based friendly options from Indian, Thai, Ethiopian, Mexican, Mediterranean, Japanese, North African, Vietnamese and Chinese cuisine

Sample Meal Plans

The following are sample meal plans from my personal experiences and from the experiences of numerous colleagues who have contributed meal plans to this chapter. All of the meal plans consist of whole plant foods and are primarily common allergen-free as well. They are nutrient-dense and focused on high net gain nutrition, not total calories at all costs, like many athletes are used to consuming.

These meal plans are designed to be guidelines and examples. Chances are good that these meal plans will yield more nutrition than you are currently consuming because they don't have refined or processed foods, fillers, or empty calories and are very nutrient-dense. You can follow them exactly, or you can alter them based on your own food preferences, the foods you have access to, based on your own unique health and fitness goals. You may require more or fewer calories based on your BMR, and ultimately based on your very specific goals, which you have established back when you read Chapter Two. You are also advised to consult your own nutritionist, physician, or health expert before starting a new nutrition program inspired by the suggestions in this chapter.

There will be numerous samples containing a variety of foods from international entrees to exotic fruits, to very common foods you'll find in essentially any major metropolitan grocery store worldwide. I hope you find some meal plans that resonate with you, and that provide a baseline from which to work as you formulate your nutritional approach to achieve your goals. Be forewarned that some meal plans are deceptively simple. That is by design. Good nutrition doesn't have to be complicated. It can still be exotic, full of flavor and incredibly satisfying, but it can also be amazingly practical, simple, and effective. I tend to focus on the latter. I am not a chef, I am not a foodie, and I am not a culinary expert, but I do know how to fuel my body to achieve the results I am looking for, be it fat-loss, muscle gain, or something else like strength gain, or incredible endurance. It doesn't mean I don't appreciate tantalizing plant-based culinary delights, and I do indulge in exotic entrees at high-end plant-based restaurants in San Francisco, Vancouver, New York City, Los Angeles, Toronto, Asheville, Portland, and other plant-based cuisine hot spots, but that is not the foundation for which my nutritional desires are based, and I am going out on a limb to assume it's not for most of you either. Whatever your nutritional desires, I hope you find some of the following sample meal plans to be helpful, even if they are deceptively simple.

This is what a typical day looks like for me:

Breakfast

- Water
- A few pieces of whole fruit
- A bowl of oats with berries or other fruit
- A green smoothie made from green leafy vegetables, water, and fruit

Snack

- A few pieces of whole fruit
- Vegetables and hummus
- Yerba Mate drink

Lunch

- International cuisine such as Thai, Indian, or Mexican
- Small green salad
- Water

Snack

- A few pieces of whole fruit
- A fruit, nut and seed bar
- Water

Dinner

- Potatoes, lentils, beans, brown rice, quinoa or other starchy complex carbohydrate food
- Green salad
- International cuisine
- Water

Snack

- A few pieces of whole fruit
- A fruit, nut and seed bar
- Occasionally something heavy such as potatoes, beans, lentils

The usual variations include more salad greens as snacks, foods such as plant-based sushi (avocado and vegetable rolls) as snacks or primary meals, occasionally nuts and seeds, and other types of international foods. I traditionally keep potatoes, yams, beans, lentils, brown rice, and quinoa as my foundational staples and include salad greens, vegetables, fruits, nuts and seeds and complimentary foods that add flavor, texture, variety and nutrition to the main courses of my meals. Most of my snacks are fruit-based, comprised of the following: Bananas, oranges, apples, grapes, raspberries, blueberries, blackberries, strawberries, melons, tangerines, pears, mangos, and whatever is in season at the time. Cherries are an all-time favorite fruit of mine, with lychee, mango, watermelon, and persimmons all making my list of preferred fruits when in season. For convenience sake, I often snack on fruit, nut and seed bars for quick dense calories before, during or after workouts, and when traveling.

Ultimately, I want to eat nutrient-dense foods as often as possible, therefore salad greens are added to most of my main courses and fruits are consumed throughout the day, including pre, post, and often during muscle-building workouts. Starchy complex carbohydrates always provide me with the most fuel. Those are the true staples of my diet, with fruit and yams and potatoes being favorite foods, and Thai, Indian, and Mexican being my absolute preferred foods based on diversity of nutrition, overall taste, flavor, enjoyment, and the satiation that comes from these amazing meals.

Now that you know what I am eating day in and day out to fuel what is arguably my most efficient and athletically complete physique I have had, I will turn the meal plan recommendations over to my colleagues who have a much more intricate approach to food preparation than my primitive nutrition plans. The best part is, whether you follow my approach or their approaches, as long as your true nutrition foundation is made up of plant-based whole foods with roughly a 70/15/15 intake, you are well on your way to nutrition, health and athletic success!

A week's worth of healthy, whole-food meal plans by Holistic Health Coach, Elena Kulakovska

kulhealthyyou.com

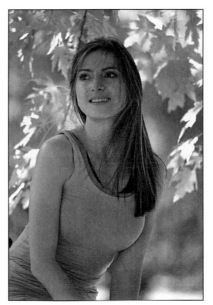

Elena Kulakovska

Elena is a certified holistic health coach helping athletes improve their fitness through nutrition. Through individually tailored programs, she also helps people make healthier lifestyle choices that stick for the long term.

1. Daily Menu for Athletes

Breakfast:

Smoothie

   3 cups collard greens

   2 tbsp ground flaxseed

   1 cup blueberries

   1 banana (frozen or fresh)

   1/4 cup pumpkin seeds

   1 cup water

Blend all ingredients in Vitamix or other high power blender until smooth. Enjoy.

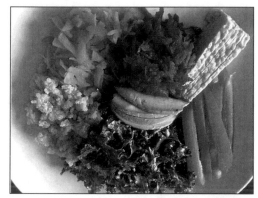

Photo by Elena Kulakovska

Lunch:

Salad with Tempeh

   3 cups mixed greens

   2 cups romaine lettuce

   1 avocado

   1 cup carrots (grated)

   1/2 cup raw beets (grated)

   1/2 sweet red pepper (diced)

   1 cup quinoa (cooked)

   1/2 block tempeh

Salad dressing (mix 2 tbsp tahini + 2 tbsp apple cider vinegar + pinch of sea salt)

Snack:

- 1 apple
- 1 slice sprouted grain bread
- 2 tsp raw almond butter

Dinner:

Rainbow Bowl

- 2 cups raw broccoli (chopped)
- 2 raw sweet red peppers (chopped)
- 1/2 cup hummus
- 3 cups kale (cooked)
- 2 cups shiitake mushrooms (cooked)
- 1/2 cup peas (cooked)
- 1/4 cup raw cashews (soaked in water for 6-8 hours)
- 1/2 cup almond milk
- 1 tbsp sesame seeds
- 1 cup wild rice (cooked)
- 3 cups kabocha squash (baked)

In a pan lightly sauté kale, shiitake mushrooms and peas in *cashew cream sauce

*To prepare the cashew cream sauce, place the soaked cashews, almond milk, and nutritional yeast flakes in a blender, and blend until smooth.

In a bowl, mix raw broccoli with sweet red pepper, hummus, sautéed kale, shiitake mushrooms, and peas. Top with sesame seeds and serve over wild rice and baked Kabocha squash.

Snack:

Date Rolls

- 3 Medjool dates
- 1/4 cup hemp seeds
- 2 tbsp shredded coconut

Process all ingredients in a food processor and form into small rolls.

2. Daily Menu for Athletes

Breakfast:

Oatmeal and Sprouted Grain Bread
with Raw Almond Butter

1 cup oatmeal (cooked)

2 tbsp ground flaxseeds

1/4 cup sunflower seeds

1 apple (sliced)

1 banana (sliced)

1/2 tsp cinnamon

Plus:

1 slice sprouted grain bread

2 tbsp raw almond butter

For the oatmeal, mix in a bowl cooked oatmeal with flaxseed and sunflower seeds, top with apple and banana slices and sprinkle with cinnamon. Spread 2 tbsp almond butter on a slice of sprouted grain bread.

Lunch:

Soup and Salad

Mixed greens salad topped with chickpeas, avocado, tomato, red pepper, tempeh, and creamy blueberry salad dressing (cashews, sunflower seeds, fresh blueberries, vinegar)

1 serving of vegetable split pea soup (vegetable stock, mushrooms, parsnips, leeks, split peas, green collards, broccoli rabe, almond butter, basil, dill, thyme, nutritional yeast)

For Salad:

5 cups mixed greens

1 tomato

1 avocado

1/2 cup chickpeas (cooked)

1 cup sweet red pepper (diced)

1/4 block tempeh

For Soup (makes 2 servings):
   2 cups vegetable stock
   1/2 cup mushrooms
   1/4 cup carrots
   1/2 cup leeks
   1/2 cup split peas
   1/2 cup collard greens
   1/2 cup broccoli rabe
   2 tbsp almond butter
   1 tbsp nutritional yeast flakes

Snack:

Smoothie

   2 cups spinach
   2 cups kale
   1 banana
   1 cup pineapple (diced)
   1 cup blueberries
   1/4 almonds
   1 cup water

Blend all ingredients in Vitamix or other high power blender until smooth. Enjoy.

Dinner:

In a bowl, mix steamed broccoli with zucchini, tomato, cooked lentils, cooked mushrooms, and nutritional yeast, and top over quinoa. Serve alongside baked sweet potato.
   3 cups broccoli (steamed)
   1/2 cup lentils (cooked)
   1/2 cup mushrooms (cooked)
   1 tbsp nutritional yeast
   1 cup quinoa (cooked)
   1 zucchini (chopped)
   1 tomato
   1 baked sweet potato

Snack:

Slices of apple (serve dipped in nut butter, with cinnamon sprinkled over top)

    1 apple

    2 tbsp raw cashew butter

    Dash of cinnamon

3. Daily Menu for Athletes

Breakfast:

PB & J Smoothie

    3 cups spinach

    1 cup frozen or fresh raspberries

    2 stalks celery

    2 tbsp almond butter

    2 Medjool dates

    1 cup almond milk (unsweetened)

Blend all ingredients in Vitamix or other high power blender until smooth. Enjoy.

Lunch:

Quinoa Avocado Wrap

    1 cup quinoa (cooked)

    1 sprouted tortilla

    1/2 avocado

    1 tomato

    1 cucumber

    1 large carrot

    1/2 tsp cayenne pepper

    1 tbsp dulse flakes (optional) - highly beneficial to athletes as it helps replenish electrolytes

    3 tbsp tahini

    2 tbsp apple cider vinegar

    Salad dressing (mix 2 tbsp tahini + 2 tbsp apple cider vinegar + pinch of sea salt)

Slice avocado, tomatoes, cucumber, and grate carrot. Place, along with dulse and quinoa, on tortilla. Drizzle salad dressing over top. Roll up, tucking ends in so the wrap is secure. Cut into pieces if desired.

Snack:

Slices of apple

(serve dipped in nut butter, with cinnamon sprinkled over top)

>1 apple
>
>2 tbsp nut butter
>
>Dash of cinnamon

Dinner:

Quinoa Bowl

>1 cup quinoa (cooked)
>
>1/3 cup organic edamame (cooked)
>
>1/2 cup almond milk
>
>1/4 cup shelled hemp seeds (can substitute pumpkin seeds if hemp seeds are not available)
>
>1/4 cup nutritional yeast
>
>1 tbsp Dijon mustard
>
>1/2 tsp turmeric
>
>1 tbsp lemon juice
>
>Black pepper to taste
>
>3/4 cups steamed and chopped sweet potato
>
>2 cups finely chopped raw kale

1) To make the sauce, place the almond milk, hemp, nutritional yeast, mustard, turmeric, lemon, and salt and pepper in a high-speed blender and blend until smooth and creamy. Add about 1/2 cup sauce to the quinoa, and stir to combine.

2) Heat up quinoa on medium heat. Add the chopped sweet potato, cooked edamame and kale to the quinoa, and stir for a few minutes, until the kale wilts and everything is hot. At this point, if the quinoa isn't as creamy as you'd like, add more sauce. If it's perfect, then simply save the remaining sauce for another meal.

3) Top the dish with more nutritional yeast or hemp seeds, if desired, and serve.

Snack:

Ice-No-Cream

1 frozen banana

1 tsp raw cacao powder

1/3 cup almond milk

Blend everything in a high-speed blender until smooth. Enjoy as soft serve ice cream.

4. Daily Menu for Athletes

Breakfast:

Smoothie

1/2 cup water

1/2 almond milk

4 ice cubes

1 Medjool date

1 cup frozen or fresh mango

Juice of 1 lime

2 tbsp ground flaxseeds

Blend all ingredients in Vitamix or other high power blender until smooth. Enjoy.

Lunch:

Quinoa and Lentil Salad

2 cups mixed greens

1 cup quinoa (cooked)

1/2 large cucumber, diced

1 small bell pepper, diced

1/2 cup lentils (cooked)

1/2 cup fresh parsley, chopped

For the vinaigrette:

1/4 cup apple cider vinegar

1/3 cup fresh squeezed orange juice

1 tbsp Dijon mustard

1 clove garlic, diced

1 tsp cumin

Salt and pepper to taste

Mix quinoa with chopped vegetables, lentils and parsley. Whisk dressing ingredients, add to the salad, and serve.

Snack:

Celery and Carrot Sticks with Hummus

2 stalks celery (cut into 2 inch sticks)

2 large carrots (cut into 2 inch sticks)

3 tbsp hummus

Dinner:

Massaged Kale and Avocado Salad, served with Brown Rice

1 head kale, shredded

1 avocado, chopped

2 tbsp lemon juice

1 tsp sea salt

*1/2 tsp dulse flakes (optional) - highly beneficial to athletes as it helps replenish electrolytes

1/2 tsp cayenne

1 cup red bell pepper, diced

1 cup brown rice (cooked)

In a mixing bowl, toss all ingredients (except for the brown rice), squeezing as you mix (hence the title word "massaged") to wilt the kale and cream the avocado. Add the diced red bell pepper and mix well. Serve immediately with 1 cup of brown rice.

* Dulse is a sea vegetable that provides the perfect mineral balance in a natural form and is an excellent source of the minerals and trace elements we need daily for optimal health, and especially during athletic training.

Snack:

Sea-Salted Popcorn

4 cups organic popcorn

(the only ingredients should be organic corn and sea salt)

5. Daily Menu for Athletes

Breakfast:

Apple Oat Smoothie

1 cup oatmeal (cooked)

2 tbsp almond butter

1 apple (chopped)

1/4 tsp nutmeg

1 tsp cinnamon

1/2 cup ice

1 cup almond milk (unsweetened)

A few drops of vanilla extract (optional)

Blend all ingredients in Vitamix or other high power blender until smooth. Enjoy.

Lunch:

Salad

3 cups mixed greens

1 cup spinach

1 avocado

1 cup tomatoes (chopped)

1/2 cup cucumber (chopped)

1/2 sweet red pepper (diced)

1 cup quinoa (cooked)

1/2 block tempeh

Salad dressing:

(mix 2 tbsp tahini + 2 tbsp apple cider vinegar + pinch of sea salt)

Snack:

Fruit and Nuts

1 apple

1/4 cup walnuts

1/4 cup raisins

Dinner:

Shiitake Mushroom, Buckwheat and Quinoa Stir Fry

Sauce:

Juice from 1 lime

2 tbsp low sodium tamari sauce

1 tsp rice wine vinegar

1/2 tsp fine ground sea salt

Juice from 1/2 navel orange

Stir Fry:

1 cup quinoa (cooked)

1 cup buckwheat (cooked)

1-2 cups shiitake mushrooms, sliced (use as many as you like)

1/4 cup cashews, chopped

1/2 red onion, diced

1 large carrot, diced

1 cup sugar snap peas, sliced into 1/2 inch pieces

3 green onions, sliced thinly

2 tbsp fresh minced ginger root

2 cloves garlic, minced

3 tbsp chopped parsley leaves

5 tbsp vegetable stock or water

Squeeze fresh lime and orange juice into a medium bowl. Add remaining sauce ingredients and stir well. Set aside.

In a skillet (or wok if you have one) heated to medium-high, cook red onion and carrots with 3 tbsp vegetable stock or water for 7 minutes. Stir often. Now, increase heat of skillet to high, add mushrooms and 2 tbsp vegetable stock or water. Stir for one minute.

Add ginger, garlic, half of your green onions and stir-fry for about 30 seconds. Add buckwheat and quinoa and stir-fry for about 1 minute. Fold in snap peas and stir-fry for 1 minute. Add sauce and fold together for 1 minute.

Serve immediately topped with chopped cashews, remaining green onions and parsley.

Snack:

Fruit and Nuts/Seeds

2 kiwis

1/4 cup pumpkin seeds

6. Daily Menu for Athletes

Breakfast:

Hemp Pear Smoothie

1 cup oatmeal (cooked)

1 cup spinach

1 tbsp hemp seeds

1 tbsp fresh ginger (chopped)

3/4 cup almond milk (unsweetened)

1 pear

1 Medjool date

Blend all ingredients in Vitamix or other high power blender until smooth. Enjoy.

Lunch:

Quinoa Hummus Wrap

1 cup quinoa (cooked)

1 sprouted tortilla

3 tbsp roasted red pepper hummus

1 tomato

1 cucumber

1 sweet red pepper

1/2 tsp cayenne pepper

1 tbsp dulse flakes (optional) - highly beneficial to athletes as it helps replenish electrolytes

3 tbsp tahini

2 tbsp apple cider vinegar

Salad dressing (mix 3 tbsp tahini + 2 tbsp apple cider vinegar + pinch of sea salt)

Spread hummus on sprouted tortilla wrap. Slice tomatoes, cucumber, and pepper. Place, along with dulse and quinoa, on tortilla. Drizzle salad dressing over top. Roll up, tucking ends in so the wrap is secure. Cut into pieces if desired.

Snack:

Ice-No-Cream

1 frozen banana

1/2 cup frozen blueberries

1/3 cup almond milk

Blend everything in a high-speed blender until smooth. Enjoy as soft serve ice cream.

Dinner:

Rainbow Bowl

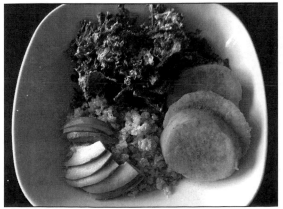

Photo by Elena Kulakovska

4 cups of mixed greens

1 roasted sweet potato, spiced with cinnamon and paprika

4 cups kale (chopped) and marinated with tahini and apple cider vinegar dressing

1/2 avocado (sliced)

1 cup cooked buckwheat

Mix all ingredients (except for the mixed greens) and arrange over the bed of mixed greens.

Snack:

Chia pudding

4 tbsp chia seeds (grounded)

1/2 almond milk (unsweetened)

1 Medjool date

Dash of cinnamon

Mash date with a little bit of the almond milk, add chia seeds and let sit for 20 minutes to form gel-like substance. Enjoy sprinkled with cinnamon.

7. Daily Menu for Athletes

Breakfast:

Ginger Hemp Green Smoothie

2 cups spinach

1 cup coconut water

1/2 cup pure water

1 banana

1/3 avocado

1 inch piece of ginger

1 tbsp hemp seeds

1 lime (peeled)

3 ice cubes

Blend all ingredients in Vitamix or other high power blender until smooth. Enjoy.

Lunch:

Collard Green Wrap with Spicy Almond Dipping Sauce

For the wrap:

    2 collard greens

    1 carrot, julienned

    1 bell pepper, julienned

    1/2 cucumber, julienned

    1/2 cup cauliflower, chopped

    1/2 avocado, sliced

For the dipping sauce:

    2 inch piece of ginger

    1 tomato

    1/4 cup fresh lemon juice

    1/4 cup almond butter

    2 cloves garlic

    1 tsp cayenne

    2 scallions, including white and about 3 inches of green

    2 tbsp orange juice

    1 tbsp tahini

1. Place 2 collard green leaves on your cutting board.

2. Place an equal amount of julienned vegetables in the center of leaf.

3. Blend all dipping sauce ingredients in a blender or food processor and drizzle on top of the veggies.

4. Roll each leaf tightly. Serve with extra dipping sauce on the side.

Snack:

    Kale Chips and veggies (celery and carrots)

Dinner:

Rainbow Bowl

2 cups of kale

2 cups of spinach

1 cup chickpeas (cooked)

1/2 cup shredded raw beets

1 baked sweet potato

1 cucumber (diced)

1/4 cup pumpkin seeds

1/4 avocado

Mix all ingredients (except for the kale and spinach) and arrange over the bed of mixed greens (kale and spinach).

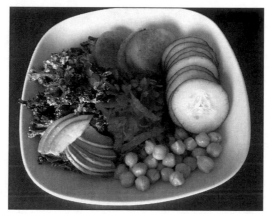

Photo by Elena Kulakovska

Snack:

Chia pudding

4 tbsp chia seeds (grounded)

1/2 cup almond milk (unsweetened)

1 Medjool date

Dash of cinnamon

Mash date with a little bit of the almond milk, add chia seeds and let sit for 20 minutes to form gel-like substance. Enjoy sprinkled with cinnamon.

Meal Plan by Plant-Based Bodybuilder, Arvid Beck

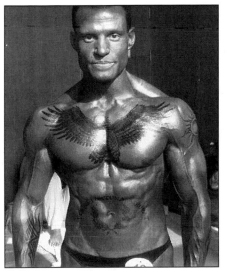

Arvid Beck

Arvid is a competitive bodybuilder from Germany. His current diet is based on whole foods, with an emphasis on carbohydrates (up to 80 percent) and little fat (usually around 10 percent), and doesn't include any protein powders. His staples are grains, legumes, vegetables, and fruits.

Exemplary Meal Plan #1: 2500 Calories

Breakfast:

Cereal-Banana-Mush

3 bananas

150 grams rolled oats

1-2 tbsp cinnamon

Liquid stevia

Lunch:

Potatoes & Baked Beans

600 grams potatoes

400 grams tomato sauce

250 grams white beans

Black pepper

Tabasco sauce

Dinner:

Salad & Fruit

200 grams mache

250 grams cherry tomatoes

1 onion

250 grams kidney beans

10 grams walnuts

2 apples

1 glass of rice milk (12 ounces)

Nutritional Value

Carbohydrates:	401 grams	(76 percent)
Fiber:	72 grams	
Protein:	76 grams	(14 percent)
Fat:	22 grams	(10 percent)

Exemplary Meal Plan #2: 2000 Calories

Breakfast:

Post-Workout Shake

450 grams banana (3 huge bananas without peel)

150 grams frozen (or fresh) blueberries

250 grams frozen spinach

10 grams highly de-oiled cacao

5 grams cinnamon

Optional: Liquid stevia (if not sweet enough)

Lunch:

Quinoa-Lentil Dish

125 grams quinoa (uncooked)

75 grams red lentils (uncooked)

Small amount of low sodium soy sauce

2 tbsp of mango chutney

Curry powder

Dinner:

Salad & Fruit

150 grams field salad

500 grams tomatoes

500 grams carrots

50 grams wheat germ

15 grams chia seeds

2 oranges

Nutritional Value

Carbohydrates:	344 grams	(70 percent)
Fiber:	85 grams	
Protein:	87 grams	(18 percent)
Fat:	25 grams	(12 percent)

– CHAPTER 9 –

Exercises to get Big and Ripped

> *"I've never really viewed myself as particularly talented.*
> *Where I excel is (through) ridiculous, sickening work ethic.*
> *While the other guy's sleeping, I'm working.*
> *While the other guy's eating, I'm working."*
>
> — Will Smith

A lot of people do the same exercises over and over with the same weight and number of repetitions and expect a different result. Eight-time Mr. Olympia Champion, Ronnie Coleman, has a wake-up call for you. "If you always do what you've always done, you always get what you always got." He probably wasn't the first to say that, but he was the first I heard say that, and like many things Ronnie says, it stuck with me. Though consistency can lead to adaptation and improvement, there are usually components such as a change in intensity, change in exercises, repetition range, and other factors that influence the end result. It is a good idea to do the same exercises for a few weeks to track progression to see if you're getting stronger in the same exercises performed weeks prior, but after four weeks or so of doing the same routine, it is wise to change it up. Simply going to the gym and riding the bike at the same resistance level for the same duration day after day won't do much except make you adapt to that very resistance level and duration to make it become a little bit easier over time. To really improve is to change things up in a more dramatic way. You could pedal faster, pedal harder, change the duration, change the style using circuits, incorporate other exercises into your morning stationary bike commute, and a whole host of other actions to change the way your body will adapt to the added stress.

The primary alterations you will want to make when adjusting your workout routine are:

1. Change the type of exercise
2. Change the level of intensity
3. Change the duration

These three simple factors can be combined in a number of ways. For example, if you go for a three-mile run every morning, and are not seeing the improved speed or endurance results you're looking for, here are some ways you can adjust your approach:

1. Combine running with rowing, cycling, swimming, box jumps, sprints, or some other type of exercise that will train your muscles and your heart and lungs differently.

2. Incorporate sprints into your workout. Run for a mile, sprint for 100 meters, and repeat. Or run three miles, followed by five to ten 100-meter sprints after your primary workout.

3. Run four miles, and build up to five miles, six, and beyond.

Additionally, you can alter the number of workouts per week, change your training style, including minor changes such as new shoes in the example above, and new gloves, wider grips, drop sets, super sets, rest pauses, and other alterations, when referring to weight training. You can change the time of day when you exercise, alter the foods you eat pre- and post-workout, train with a partner, group or team, rather than on your own, or vice versa, and many more variations what will all have some sort of impact on your end result.

Rather than sticking with the same old routine that has left you where you are now, I suggest you mix it up by turning things up a notch to get where you want to be. The following are some examples for you to examine and incorporate into your own exercise routine, if they are of interest to you. Remember, if it isn't fun, you probably won't do it, so pick the exercises that seem most enjoyable and perform them with enthusiasm and effort with a specific end result in mind.

Fat-burning cardiovascular exercises

These exercises should be performed on an empty stomach first thing in the morning to get shredded.

- Walking
- Jogging
- Running
- Sprinting
- Hiking
- Swimming
- Cycling
- Rowing
- Stair climbing
- Jumping
- Total body exercises (like Burpees)
- CrossFit
- High Intensity Interval Training
- Circuit training
- Handball or racquet sports
- Any team or individual sport involving running, rowing, swimming or cycling

Strength-building exercises to put on muscle

- Squats
- Deadlifts
- Bench press
- Overhead press
- Lunges
- Pull-ups
- Dips
- Shrugs
- Rack pulls
- Push-ups

- T-bar rows
- Bicep curls
- Skull crushers
- Olympic lifts
- Other free weight, compound exercises

Alterations to the standard lifts

Combined with the exercises listed above, you can incorporate the following:

- Low reps
- High reps
- Slow reps
- Partial reps
- Assisted reps
- 1-rep max
- Super sets
- Drop sets
- Negatives (eccentric contractions)
- Narrow grip
- Wide grip
- Neutral grip
- Reverse grip
- Rest pause
- Twenty-ones
- Pyramids

By changing the style that you perform these exercises, you change the impact it has on your body, and you can break through from your regular routine to advance with new gains. When you do this over time, you are bound to see results.

Additionally, you can change the level of intensity performed in each exercise, from fasted cardiovascular training first thing in the morning, to explosive compound, free-weight exercises. Some of those changes might look like this:

- High Intensity Training (HIT)
- High Intensity Interval Training (HIIT)
- 30 seconds on, 30 seconds off
- Increasing level of intensity in a pyramid, working your way up and back down, cycling your level of energy expenditure, changing by the minute

The following is a week's worth of sample exercises, followed by numerous options for additional workouts for set muscle groups. The exercises listed below emphasize training one or two muscle groups per day, in a muscle-building routine designed to exhaust specific muscle groups and allow them long rest periods to recover and grow. You can do total body workouts all you want, and some of those programs will be listed in this chapter as well, and your body may respond well to them. I like total body workouts, but my bodybuilding experience tells me that the following approach of targeting specific muscle groups for an entire workout is an effective one for building quality muscle. I like P90X and CrossFit as much as the next person, and my experience with those genres of training, tells me that they will surely make you very fit. To really build significant muscle and strength though, a more targeted and deliberate approach to training for muscle size is usually required. Not that total body training such as the programs mentioned above won't build muscle, I just don't believe they are as effective as focusing on one or two muscle groups a day using the best compound, free-weight exercises to elicit the greatest return on investment. Total body exercises are excellent for burning fat, getting toned, building up endurance and core strength and getting ripped. I just don't believe that helps you build as much muscle as a tailor-made approach to building muscle such as the ones I will outline in the workouts below.

When we take the time to dedicate an entire workout to training one or two muscle groups, we exercise those muscles more thoroughly and completely than we would in a more casual total body workout. Follow the guidelines listed below to put on some serious muscle. If you stick with a specific routine for four weeks, you should see results in strength and muscle gains in week four compared to week one. Then you can mix up your routine for another four weeks, and so on every three to six weeks, or whatever schedule is comfortable for you based on your own progression. Once you have experienced this type of muscle-building training, by all means, try total body workouts for weeks at a time and see how they compare to specific muscle-building training. Each of us responds differently to different workloads and stresses on the body, so always feel free to experiment with a variety of programs and follow the ones that resonate the most with you. Let's get shredded!

Sample Muscle-Building Workout Routines

An effective muscle-building schedule:

Week 1:

Monday = Chest/Shoulders

Tuesday = Back

Wednesday = Legs

Thursday = Rest

Friday = Arms

Saturday = Abs

Sunday = Rest

Week 2:

Monday = Chest

Tuesday = Back/Shoulders

Wednesday = Legs

Thursday = Rest

Friday = Arms

Saturday = Abs, forearms, calves

Sunday = Rest

Week 3:

> **Monday** = Chest
>
> **Tuesday** = Back
>
> **Wednesday** = Legs
>
> **Thursday** = Rest
>
> **Friday** = Arms/Shoulders
>
> **Saturday** = Abs
>
> **Sunday** = Rest

Week 4:

> **Monday** = Chest
>
> **Tuesday** = Back
>
> **Wednesday** = Legs
>
> **Thursday** = Rest
>
> **Friday** = Arms, forearms, calves
>
> **Saturday** = Abs/Shoulders
>
> **Sunday** = Rest

Primary multi-joint, compound, free weight and bodyweight muscle building exercises to choose from include:

Chest

- Flat bench press
- Incline bench press
- Decline bench press
- Flat dumbbell press
- Incline dumbbell press
- Decline dumbbell press
- Flat dumbbell flys
- Incline dumbbell flys

- Decline dumbbell flys
- Dips
- Push-ups
- Decline push-ups
- Various cables and machines as desired

Shoulders

- Barbell overhead press
- Dumbbell overhead press
- Dumbbell lateral raises
- Dumbbell front raises
- Dumbbell rear deltoid raises
- Upright rows
- Barbell shrugs
- Dumbbell shrugs
- One-arm dumbbell overhead raises
- Military press
- Various cables and machines as desired

Back

- Deadlifts
- Wide grip pull-ups
- Narrow grip pull-ups
- Neutral grip pull-ups
- T-Bar rows
- Bent-over rows
- One-arm dumbbell rows
- Rack pulls
- Lat pull-downs
- High rows

- Mid rows
- Low rows
- Various cables and machines as desired

Legs

- Squats
- One-legged squats
- Jump squats
- Lunges
- Jump lunges
- Leg press
- Hack squats
- Deadlifts
- Calf raises
- Box jumps
- Wall-sits
- Various cables and machines as desired

Arms

Biceps

- Alternating bicep curls
- Hammer curls
- Concentration curls
- Preacher curls
- Negatives (eccentric contractions)
- Reverse grip pull-ups
- Reverse grip lat pull-downs
- Various cables and machines as desired

Triceps

- Skull crushers
- Narrow grip bench press
- Overhead extensions
- One-arm overhead extensions
- Dumbbell kickbacks
- Negatives (eccentric contractions)
- Dips
- Push-ups
- Decline push-ups
- Various cables and machines as desired

Abs

- Hanging leg raises
- Hanging knee raises
- Windshield wipers
- Plank
- Weighted plank
- Lying leg raises
- Bicycle crunches
- Crunches
- Side crunches
- Weighted crunches
- Ab wheel roll-outs
- Sit ups
- Various cables and machines as desired

The Workouts

In the sample workouts listed below, I included a morning fasted cardio session in addition to a weight training session for the same day. The fasted cardio first thing in the morning is intended to help you efficiently burn fat, supporting your overall fitness goals. The weight training workouts are to help you build muscle, supporting your other fitness goals. If bulking up is your primary objective, you may consider omitting the morning cardio, or limiting it to once or twice a week, to avoid burning too many calories and getting too lean. The examples are exactly that, just samples and loose guidelines. You can follow them exactly and you'll get really fit and really strong, but you can also alter them based on your own interests, the equipment you have access to, and based on your own work ethic, desires, and objectives. You will notice that I prefer the 8-12 repetition range for most exercises, but that I also incorporate a good balance of high reps (around 20 or so) and low reps (6 or so) in most of the workouts. This is to train muscle fibers differently, and to engage in different lengths of time for individual sets. The varying repetitions may also bring about strength gains and produce muscle tone in ways that benefit your physique and your interests. Some people may respond better to high repetitions such as 25-50 reps per set, and some may respond better to really heavy weights with lower reps such as 3-5 reps per set. I try to incorporate a pretty good balance in the workouts provided.

In general, I like to warm up with 20-30 reps, and perform the 8-12 repetition range for my working sets. With my favorite exercises I like to lift especially heavy and just complete a few reps with as heavy weight as I can. Sometimes I like the burning sensation that comes from high repetition training for specific muscles such as biceps, triceps, quads, and calves. Yet other times I prefer to focus exclusively on Olympic lifts completing just 5-10 reps per set to thoroughly thrash my body. At the end of the day, I respect the diversity and benefits of high and low repetition training and incorporate both into my regular training routine. You can too, and take notice of how your body responds to varying stress levels through changes in repetition ranges. Experiment with high, mid, and low rep ranges for a few weeks and notice if one particular approach yields the best results or is the most fun. If it fits your interests, you can incorporate all three repetition ranges in a given workout and determine your own preferred range for your primary working sets.

Above all else, train intelligently with purpose and passion with specific goals in mind. Make it fun, keep it safe, and be open to learning, unafraid of asking questions from those who have been there, done that. Use your resources from local trainers to online discussion groups, to popular websites and books to help you construct the physique and health outcome you desire.

Sample Workout #1 – Chest and Shoulders

A sample workout for someone who wants to get big and ripped might look like this:

Morning

> Workout on an empty stomach (fasted cardio)
> 15-minute jog at a low level of intensity
> 15-minute cycle, varying levels of intensity to increase heart rate
> 15-minute row, rowing hard and fast every fifth minute for one minute

Afternoon/early evening

> Weight-training workout (chest and shoulders)
> 10 minutes of cardiovascular training to warm-up, such as using the stair stepper

Chest

- Push-ups x 3 sets of 20 (used as a warm-up for muscles used in workout)
- Incline bench press x 3 sets of 8-12 reps
- Dumbbell flys x 3 sets of 8-12 reps
- Dips or weighted dips x 3 sets of 6-8 reps with decline push-ups as super sets doing as many reps as possible for each set

Shoulders

- Lateral raises x 3 sets of 8-12 reps with super sets of front raises x 8-12 reps
- Overhead shoulder press x 3 sets of 8-10 reps
- Dumbbell shrugs x 6 (total) sets of 8-20 reps with a drop set after each initial set

Finish with 15 minutes on the stair stepper, stationary bike, or if the weather is pleasant, a nice jog out in the sun.

This sample workout for chest and shoulders covers 30 total sets, which is pretty high volume, but remember that three sets are for warm-ups and nine sets are either drop sets or super sets, which don't take up very much time. This entire workout can still be completed in an hour and is designed to use exclusively free weights and bodyweight exercises aiming for an approximate 8-12 rep range as an average for the entire workout (drop sets and super sets could be very low reps as the body is fatigued and is pushing hard immediately after completing the initial set).

Sample Workout #2 - Back

Morning

Workout on an empty stomach (fasted cardio)
30-minute swim (or alternative preferred cardiovascular exercise for half an hour)

Afternoon/early evening

10 minutes of cardiovascular exercise to warm-up, such as using the stair-stepper
Weight-training workout (Back)

- Lat pull-downs x 3 sets of 15-20 reps (used as a warm-up for muscles used in workout)
- Cable rows x 3 sets of 12-15 reps (used as an additional warm-up before free weights)
- Deadlifts x 3 sets of 8-12 reps
- T-Bar rows x 3 sets of 8-12 reps
- Pull-ups x 3 sets of 8-12 reps or to failure
- Bent-over rows x 3 sets of 8-12 reps

Finish with 15 minutes on the stair stepper, stationary bike, or if the weather is pleasant, a nice jog out in the sun.

Our backs are quite vulnerable and susceptible to injury so I choose to include a couple of warm-up sets with high repetitions before I go into a heavy lift such as deadlifts, T-bar rows, bent-over rows, or some other intense exercise. I highly suggest a significant warm-up plus stretching before engaging in deadlifts.

Sample Workout #3 - Legs

Morning

Workout on an empty stomach (fasted cardio)
30-minute hike
Circuit including 15 box jumps, 40 crunches, 30-second wall-sit – Repeat
    three times

Afternoon/early evening

10 minutes of cardiovascular exercise to warm-up, such as using the
    stair stepper

Weight training workout (Legs)

- Bodyweight squats x 3 sets of 30 reps (used as a warm-up for muscles used in workout)

- Barbell Squats x 3 sets of 8-12 reps

- Lunges carrying dumbbells x 8-12 reps, incorporating drop sets after each set, lowering the weight until using no weight at all

- Leg Press x 3 sets of 6-10 reps, super setting with jump lunges

- Calf raises x 3 sets of as many reps as possible until the burning sensation overcomes you (anyone who trains calves regularly knows this feeling very well)

Finish with 15 minutes on the stair stepper, stationary bike, or if the weather is pleasant, a nice jog out in the sun.

In this sample workout, we elected to focus on legs for the entire training session. There are plenty of training styles, including focusing on total body, upper lower body, core, or one or two muscle groups per workout. Since a real tough leg workout is one of the most challenging ways to train, and one of the most effective at building muscle and strength, I chose to isolate the legs for this workout.

We managed a nice hike in the morning to burn fat by exercising on an empty stomach, and also incorporated some box jumps, wall sits, and core work, knowing we would be calling upon leg and core strength for the weight training workout in the late afternoon. During the actual leg training workout to build muscle, we busted out approximately 21 sets (the number varies based on the actual number of drop sets completed), which included three initial sets of bodyweight squats to get the lower body warmed up and prepared to squat. The volume was a bit lower here and could easily be altered by adding another exercise such as leg extensions or by changing the three sets per exercise to four sets for some of them. I prefer four sets for most exercises and even five or more sets for certain exercises such as leg press. Using a three-set example allows for more different types of exercises to fit into the workout for this specific illustration. In my personal training, I might complete just three exercises total during a given workout, such as squats, leg presses, and lunges. I often like to pick the exercises that will give me the greatest return on investment and focus more time on those (such as squats) versus an isolated movement like machine hamstring curls. Clearly the compound, multi-joint, free-weight squats will help build more muscle than using a curl machine.

Sample Workout #4 - Arms

Morning

> Workout on an empty stomach (fasted cardio)
> 30-minute jog

Afternoon/early evening

> 10 minutes of cardiovascular exercise to warm-up, such as using the stair stepper
> Weight Training Workout (Arms)
> Push-ups x 3 sets of 15-25 reps (used as a warm-up for muscles used in workout)
> Cable curls x 3 sets of 15-20 reps (used as a warm-up for muscles used in workout)

Biceps

- Alternating dumbbell bicep curls x 3 sets of 8-12 reps
- Dumbbell hammer curls x 3 sets of 8-12 reps
- EZ curl narrow-grip bicep curls x 3 sets of 8-12 reps + negatives if desired

Triceps

- Skull crushers x 3 sets of 8-12 reps, superset with narrow-grip bench press
- Overhead extensions x 3 sets of 8-12 reps
- Dips x 3 sets of 8-12 reps, superset with decline push-ups if desired

Finish with 15 minutes on the stair stepper, stationary bike, or if the weather is pleasant, a nice jog out in the sun.

Training arms is a great way to get in and get out of the gym quickly, if time is something you are concerned with. Biceps and triceps are relatively small muscles; therefore, they recover quickly between sets. When training back or chest you may need to rest a couple of minutes between sets, but with your arms, you'll find sufficient recovery after just about a minute of rest, ready to go again for the next set. You can base this on actual time, using a clock or stopwatch, or determine this based on feel. I prefer the latter. I stretch or massage my arms between sets, or simply get a drink of water, record my set in my training journal, do arm circles, or even sit on a bench for a moment before going back to hammer out another set.

You might discover that training arms will require less overall time. You may spend up to 90 minutes training legs, due to long recovery periods for large muscle groups and the sheer number of reps and sets you may need to perform to include quads, hamstrings, glutes, and calves in one workout. A chest/shoulders or back workout might take 60-75 minutes to perform, whereas an arm workout could easily be completed in less than an hour. You'll still get a sufficient pump, breakdown lots of muscle tissue, and feel content with a hardcore lifting session that was only 48 minutes long. No shame in that. Carry on, my friend.

Sample Workout #5 - Abs

Morning

Workout on an empty stomach (fasted cardio)
30 minutes on the spin bike

Afternoon/early evening

10 minutes of cardiovascular exercise to warm-up, such as using the stair stepper

Weight Training Workout (Abs)

- Front crunches x 3 sets of 25 reps (used as a warm-up for muscles used in workout)
- Left side crunches x 3 sets of 25 reps (used as a warm-up for muscles used in workout)
- Right side crunches x 3 sets of 25 reps (used as a warm-up for muscles used in workout)
- Hanging leg raises x 3 sets of as many reps as possible – Superset with hanging knee raises until failure
- Plank x 3 sets for 90 seconds or until failure
- Lying leg raises x 3 sets of 20 reps
- Bicycle crunches x 3 sets of 100 reps (50 each side)

Finish with 15 minutes on the stair stepper, stationary bike, or if the weather is pleasant, a nice jog out in the sun.

If you train your abdominals appropriately, you will feel a similar level of exhaustion you will experience during or immediately following a back or chest workout. I bet you haven't experienced that sensation training abs all that often. A lot of us tend to focus on a few sets of sit-ups or crunches, a plank or two, and call it good. Abdominal training is often tacked on to the end of some other workout. For some of the same reasons we often avoid doing lunges, we avoid doing extensive abdominal training—it hurts and it isn't always loads of fun.

When was the last time you truly looked forward to doing 3-5 sets of planks for as long as possible until falling face-first on the ground, or doing hanging leg raises until your forearms, not your abs, told you it was time to call it a day? My guess is never. Rarely do we get super pumped about exercises that lead to a strong burning sensation that challenges us mentally, physically, and aerobically. Rather than just tacking abdominal training on to the end of your workout, give abdominals their own workout, or split the time evenly with some other muscle group, like you do with chest and shoulders, biceps and triceps, and quads and hamstrings.

Summary

The workouts listed above will carve out a lean and strong physique for you if you follow the routine for four to six weeks. After that length of time performing the same exercises week after week, adapting and getting stronger, it would be a good idea to change it up, incorporating new exercises, adjusting the repetition range, and forcing your body to adapt to new stresses placed upon it. As you get more comfortable with all of these free weight exercises, you might want to change up a routine every three or four weeks, allowing just enough time to achieve noticeable strength gains in the same exercises week after week before creating a new baseline with different exercises. If you maintain the same exact routine for too long, say a couple of months with no change, you will likely hit a few plateaus, lose interest, notice longer periods between measurable improvements, and it will likely compel you to seek out a new approach. Likewise, if you're really adventurous you could change your workout routine every week, or even every day. Do what works for you, do what you enjoy, and work hard to reach your goals.

Review the lists of exercises, training styles, and workout routines listed above, and evaluate the approaches to fat-loss and muscle building (from the previous chapters) and determine what best fits into your schedule, based on your specific goals.

Consider the following additional samples for ways you can alter your weight training workouts, using a combination of free weights, machines, and cables to achieve the gains you are looking to experience. I selected the repetition range of 8-12 because it is the most commonly performed by weight lifters. It doesn't mean you need to stick within this range. There are various benefits from training with lower repetitions (some train with a 1-rep max approach for strength), as well as training with higher repetitions. As mentioned earlier, my exercise sets routinely range between three and thirty repetitions, sometimes during the same workout. Some exercises are such powerful movements I naturally want to do a lower amount of reps with heavy weights. Exercises such as T-bar rows, bench press, leg press, and power cleans come to mind. Squats and deadlifts might fit into this category for many as well. Other exercises, I naturally want to do a lot of reps for, including calf raises, biceps and triceps exercises, leg extensions, and most abdominal movements. Your personal rep range many vary based on your goals, your preferences, the equipment you have available, and numerous other factors from your range of motion/flexibility to nagging injuries or other limitations, to your level of aerobic conditioning.

Determine your own personal desired repetition range and incorporate many of the following exercises into your routine. I list the 15-20 repetition range for most warm-up exercises and the 8-12 repetition range for most working sets in the examples below because that is what I follow, and it is a common approach among many lifters. If you are a beginner or do not have a specific range you work within, 8-12 repetitions is a standard range that most people would benefit from. These daily workouts are just samples. You can follow them directly or incorporate whichever aspects you like from each one into your current training program. As usual, if you have your own personal trainer, lifting coach, or other fitness instructor, consult with them and see how these programs fit in with their objectives for you, based on your specific fitness goals. Train hard, use good form, be safe, and have fun!

Additional Sample Muscle-Building Workouts

Sample Chest Workout #1

Warm-up (10 minutes)

Stair stepper, stationary bike, treadmill, jogging, or some other type of cardiovascular exercise to get blood flowing and joints and muscles warmed up.

- Push-ups x 3 sets of 20 reps (used as an additional warm-up before free weights)
- Incline barbell bench press x 3 sets of 8-12 reps
- Flat dumbbell press x 3 sets of 8-12 reps
- Decline barbell bench press x 3 sets of 8-12 reps
- Dumbbell flys x 3 sets of 8-12 reps
- Dips x 3 sets of 8-12 reps

Total = 18 sets

Finish with 15 minutes on the stair stepper, stationary bike, or if the weather is pleasant, a nice jog out in the sun.

Follow workout with an emphasis on recovery foods, high in quality muscle-building nutrition, such as fruits, starches, greens, vegetables, legumes, nuts and seeds.

Sample Chest Workout #2

Warm-up (10 minutes)

Stair stepper, stationary bike, treadmill, jogging, or some other type of cardiovascular exercise to get blood flowing and joints and muscles warmed up.

- Push-ups x 3 sets of 20 reps (used as an additional warm-up before free weights)
- Incline dumbbell press x 3 sets of 8-12 reps
- Flat dumbbell press x 3 sets of 8-12 reps
- Decline barbell bench press x 3 sets of 8-12 reps
- Incline dumbbell flys x 3 sets of 8-12 reps
- High pulley cable cross-overs x 3 sets of 8-12 reps
- Low pulley cable cross-overs x 3 sets of 8-12 reps

Total = 21 sets

Finish with 15 minutes on the stair stepper, stationary bike, or if the weather is pleasant, a nice jog out in the sun.

Follow workout with an emphasis on recovery foods, high in quality muscle-building nutrition, such as fruits, starches, greens, vegetables, legumes, nuts and seeds.

Sample Shoulder Workout #1

Warm-up (10 minutes)

Stair stepper, stationary bike, treadmill, jogging or some other type of cardiovascular exercise to get blood flowing and joints and muscles warmed up.

- Push-ups x 3 sets of 20 reps (used as an additional warm-up before free weights)
- Lateral dumbbell raises x 3 sets of 8-12 reps
- Front dumbbell raises x 3 sets of 8-12 reps

- Upright rows x 3 sets of 8-12 reps
- Overhead barbell press x 3 sets of 8-12 reps
- Behind the back barbell shrugs x 3 sets of 8-12 reps

Total = 18 sets

Finish with 15 minutes on the stair stepper, stationary bike, or if the weather is pleasant, a nice jog out in the sun.

Follow workout with an emphasis on recovery foods, high in quality muscle-building nutrition, such as fruits, starches, greens, vegetables, legumes nuts and seeds.

Sample Shoulder Workout #2

Warm-up (10 minutes)

Stair stepper, stationary bike, treadmill, jogging or some other type of cardiovascular exercise to get blood flowing and joints and muscles warmed up.

- Push-ups x 3 sets of 20 reps (used as an additional warm-up before free weights)
- Low pulley cable cross-over lateral/rear deltoid raises x 3 sets of 8-12 sets
- Overhead dumbbell press x 3 sets of 8-12 reps
- One-arm dumbbell presses from floor x 3 sets of 8-12 reps
- Dumbbell shrugs x 3 sets of 8-12 reps
- Angled incline seated shoulder front deltoid raises x 3 sets of 8-12 reps

Total = 18 sets

Finish with 15 minutes on the stair stepper, stationary bike, or if the weather is pleasant, a nice jog out in the sun.

Follow workout with an emphasis on recovery foods, high in quality muscle-building nutrition, such as fruits, starches, greens, vegetables, legumes, nuts and seeds.

Sample Back Workout #1

Warm-up (10 minutes)

Stair stepper, stationary bike, treadmill, jogging, or some other type of cardiovascular exercise to get blood flowing and joints and muscles warmed up.

- Lat pull-downs x 3 sets of 15-20 reps (used as a warm-up for muscles used in workout)
- Machine rows x 3 sets of 12-15 reps (used as an additional warm-up before free weights)
- Pull-ups x 3 sets of 8-12 reps or to failure
- Rack pulls x 3 sets of 8-12 reps
- T-bar rows x 3 sets of 8-12 reps
- One-arm dumbbell rows x 3 sets of 8-12 reps

Total = 18 sets

Finish with 15 minutes on the stair stepper, stationary bike, or if the weather is pleasant, a nice jog out in the sun.

Follow workout with an emphasis on recovery foods, high in quality muscle-building nutrition, such as fruits, starches, greens, vegetables, legumes, nuts and seeds.

Sample Back Workout #2

Warm-up (10 minutes)

Stair stepper, stationary bike, treadmill, jogging, or some other type of cardiovascular exercise to get blood flowing and joints and muscles warmed up.

- Cable rows x 3 sets of 15-20 reps (used as an additional warm-up before free weights)
- Cable pull-downs x 3 sets of 12-15 reps (used as an additional warm-up before free weights)
- Rack pulls x 4 sets of 8-12 reps

- Deadlifts x 4 sets of 8-12 reps
- T-bar rows x 4 sets of 8-12 reps
- Pull-ups x 4 sets of 8-12 reps

Total = 22 sets

Finish with 15 minutes on the stair stepper, stationary bike, or if the weather is pleasant, a nice jog out in the sun.

Follow workout with an emphasis on recovery foods, high in quality muscle-building nutrition, such as fruits, starches, greens, vegetables, legumes, nuts and seeds.

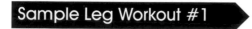

Sample Leg Workout #1

Warm-up (10 minutes)

Stair stepper, stationary bike, treadmill, jogging, or some other type of cardiovascular exercise to get blood flowing and joints and muscles warmed up.

- Bodyweight squats x 3 sets of 30 reps (used as a warm-up for muscles used in workout)
- Front squats x 3 sets of 8-12 reps
- Hack squats x 3 sets of 8-12 reps
- Leg press x 3 sets of 6-10 reps, super setting with jump lunges
- Toe presses on leg press machine x 3 sets of as many reps as possible until the burning sensation overcomes you (anyone who trains calves regularly knows this feeling very well).

Total = 18 sets

Finish with 15 minutes on the stair stepper, stationary bike, or if the weather is pleasant, a nice jog out in the sun.

Follow workout with an emphasis on recovery foods, high in quality muscle-building nutrition, such as fruits, starches, greens, vegetables, legumes, nuts and seeds.

Sample Leg Workout #2

Warm-up (10 minutes)

Stair stepper, stationary bike, treadmill, jogging, or some other type of cardiovascular exercise to get blood flowing and joints and muscles warmed up.

- Bodyweight squats x 3 sets of 30 reps (used as a warm-up for muscles used in workout)
- Barbell squats x 3 sets of 8-12 reps
- Leg extensions x 3 sets of 8-12 reps
- Lying hamstring curls x 3 sets of 8-12 reps
- Deadlifts x 3 sets of 8-12 reps
- Standing calf raises x 3 sets of as many reps as possible until the burning sensation overcomes you (anyone who trains calves regularly knows this feeling very well).
- Seated toe presses x 3 sets of as many reps as possible until the burning sensation overcomes you (anyone who trains calves regularly knows this feeling very well).

Total = 21 sets

Finish with 15 minutes on the stair stepper, stationary bike, or if the weather is pleasant, a nice jog out in the sun.

Follow workout with an emphasis on recovery foods, high in quality muscle-building nutrition, such as fruits, starches, greens, vegetables, legumes, nuts and seeds.

Sample Arm Workout #1

Push-ups x 3 sets of 15-25 reps (used as a warm-up for muscles used in workout)

Cable curls x 3 sets of 15-20 reps (used as a warm-up for muscles used in workout)

Biceps

- Alternating dumbbell bicep curls x 3 sets of 8-12 reps
- Dumbbell hammer curls x 3 sets of 8-12 reps
- EZ curl narrow-grip bicep curls x 3 sets of 8-12 reps

Triceps

- Skull crushers x 3 sets of 8-12 reps
- Overhead extensions x 3 sets of 8-12 reps
- Dips x 3 sets of 8-12 reps

Total = 24 sets

Finish with 15 minutes on the stair stepper, stationary bike, or if the weather is pleasant, a nice jog out in the sun.

Follow workout with an emphasis on recovery foods, high in quality muscle-building nutrition, such as fruits, starches, greens, vegetables, legumes, nuts and seeds.

Sample Arm Workout #2

Push-ups x 3 sets of 15-25 reps (used as a warm-up for muscles used in workout)

Machine curls x 3 sets of 15-20 reps (used as a warm-up for muscles used in workout)

Biceps

- One arm dumbbell concentration curls x 3 sets of 8-12 reps
- EZ curl preacher curls x 3 sets of 8-12 reps
- Two arm straight bar bicep curls x 3 sets of 8-12 reps

Triceps

- Narrow-grip bench press x 3 sets of 8-12 reps
- Decline push-ups with neutral grip x 3 sets of 8-12 reps
- Dumbbell kickbacks x 3 sets of 8-12 reps

Total = 24 sets

Finish with 15 minutes on the stair stepper, stationary bike, or if the weather is pleasant, a nice jog out in the sun.

Follow workout with an emphasis on recovery foods, high in quality muscle-building nutrition, such as fruits, starches, greens, vegetables, legumes, nuts and seeds.

Sample Abdominal Workout #1

- Front crunches x 3 sets of 25 reps (used as a warm-up for muscles used in workout)
- Left side crunches x 3 sets of 25 reps (used as a warm-up for muscles used in workout)
- Right side crunches x 3 sets of 25 reps (used as a warm-up for muscles used in workout)
- Cable crunches x 3 sets of 15-20 reps
- Weighted decline sit-ups x 3 sets of 8-12 reps
- Hanging knee raises to the front, left and right sides, x 3 sets of 10-15 reps
- Lying leg raises x 3 sets of 15-20 reps

Total = 21 sets

Finish with 15 minutes on the stair stepper, stationary bike, or if the weather is pleasant, a nice jog out in the sun.

Follow workout with an emphasis on recovery foods, high in quality muscle-building nutrition, such as fruits, starches, greens, vegetables, legumes, nuts and seeds.

Sample Abdominal Workout #2

- Front crunches x 3 sets of 25 reps (used as a warm-up for muscles used in workout)

- Left side crunches x 3 sets of 25 reps (used as a warm-up for muscles used in workout)

- Right side crunches x 3 sets of 25 reps (used as a warm-up for muscles used in workout)

- Hanging leg raises x 3 sets of as many reps as possible

- Weighted abdominal crunch machine x 3 sets of 15-20 reps

- Medicine ball partner sit-ups x 3 sets x as many reps as possible

- Cable sledge hammer/axe swings x 3 sets of 15-20 reps per side

- Plank x 3 sets until failure

Total = 24 sets

Finish with 15 minutes on the stair stepper, stationary bike, or if the weather is pleasant, a nice jog out in the sun.

Follow workout with an emphasis on recovery foods, high in quality muscle-building nutrition, such as fruits, starches, greens, vegetables, legumes, nuts and seeds.

Summary

If you have questions about how to complete any of the exercises listed, please use the wonderful resources found on the Internet to search for photos, videos, descriptions, and demonstrations. I'm not going to leave you hanging, on your own to seek this information out. I have recruited my favorite vegan fitness model, Mindy Collette, to join me in demonstrating some key exercises that make up the core of the various exercise programs outlined in this chapter. I hope these photo demonstrations help you perform the exercises with a greater level of confidence and understanding.

We opted to demonstrate the exercises that are perhaps the least common of the exercises listed, making the assumption that many of you are familiar with the basics such as a standard bench press, push-up, and squat. Though many are familiar with a standard push-up, an exercise like a skull crusher or T-bar row may be more foreign.

These photos are listed roughly in the order of how they are listed in this chapter:

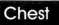 **Incline Barbell Bench Press**

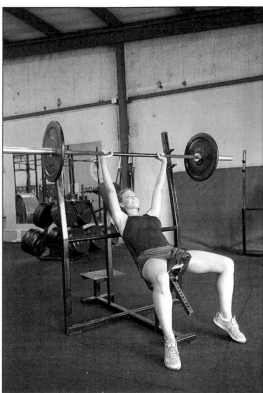

Incline Barbell Bench Press - Start

Incline Barbell Bench Press - Finish

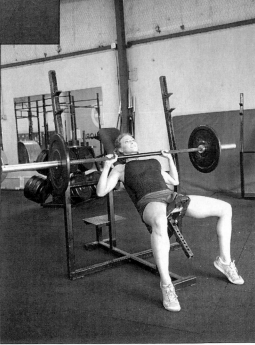

Chest

Dumbbell Flys

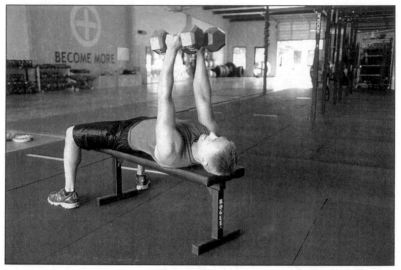

Dumbbell Flys - Start

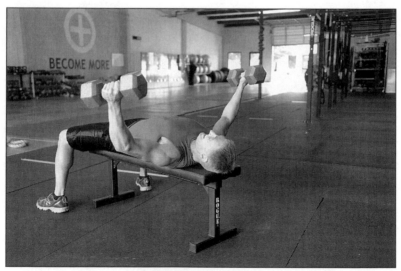

Dumbbell Flys - Finish

Chest **Dips**

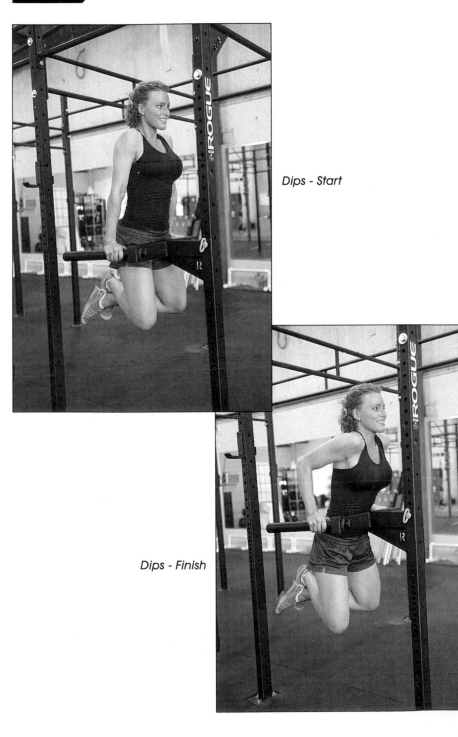

Dips - Start

Dips - Finish

Chest   **Decline Push-ups**

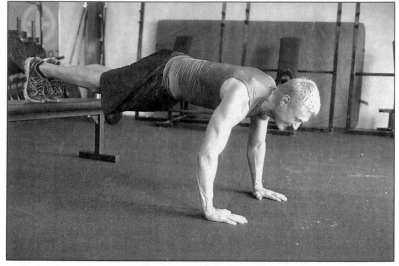

Decline Push-ups - Start

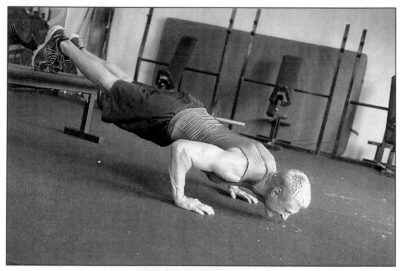

Decline Push-ups - Finish

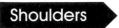 **Shoulders** **Barbell Overhead Press**

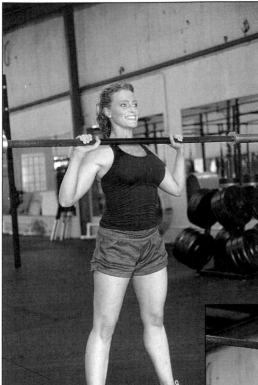

Barbell Overhead Press - Start

Barbell Overhead Press - Finish

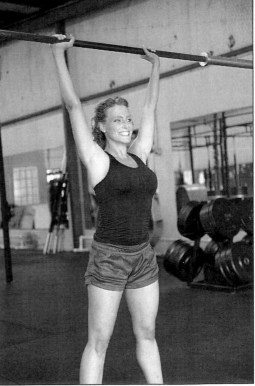

Shoulders **Dumbbell Shrugs**

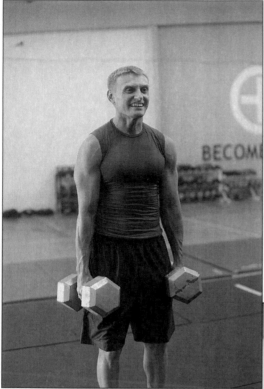

Dumbbell Shrugs - Start

Dumbbell Shrugs - Finish

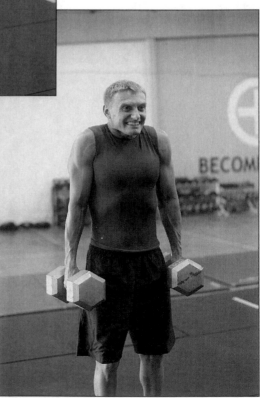

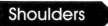
Shoulders

Upright Rows

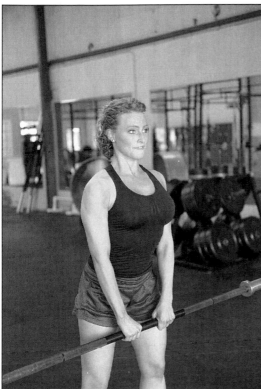

Barbell Upright Rows - Start

Barbell Upright Rows - Finish

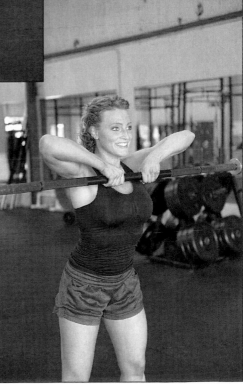

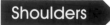 **Seated Angled Dumbbell Raises**

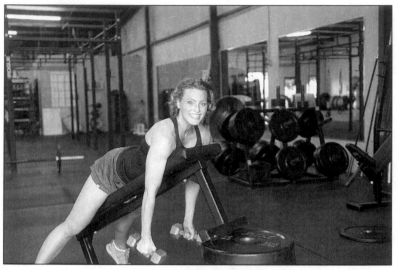

Angled Dumbbell Shoulder Raises - Start

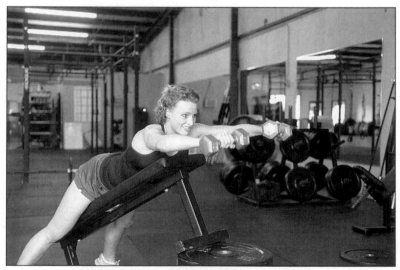

Angled Dumbbell Shoulder Raises - Finish

Back

T-bar Rows

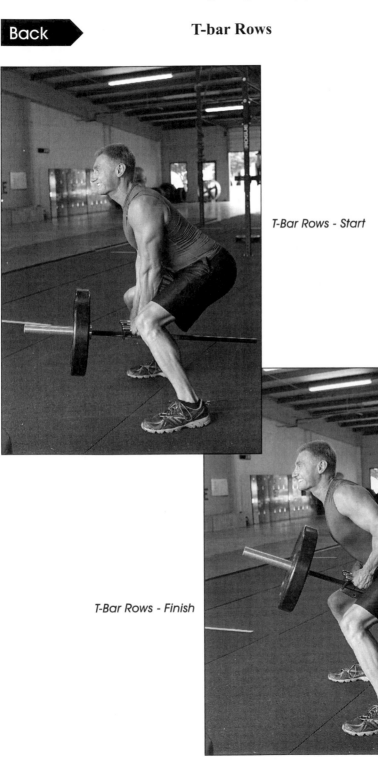

T-Bar Rows - Start

T-Bar Rows - Finish

Back

One-arm Dumbbell Rows

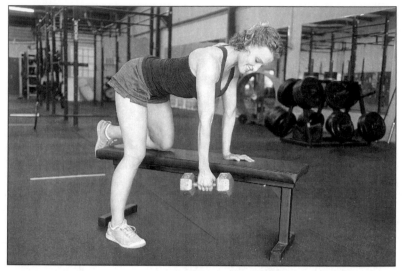

One-arm Dumbbell Rows - Start

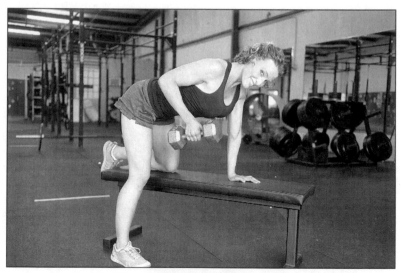

One-arm Dumbbell Rows - Finish

Back

Rack Pulls

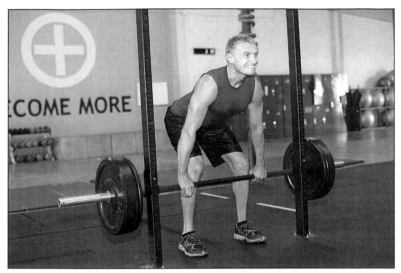

Rack Pulls - Start

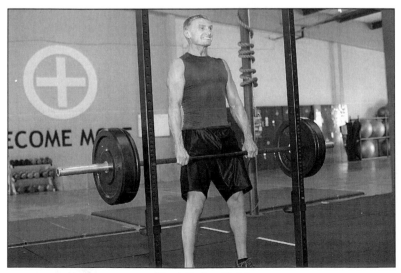

Rack Pulls - Finish

Back   **Bent-over Rows**

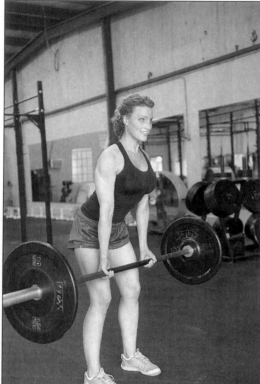

Bent-over Rows - Start

Bent-over Rows - Finish

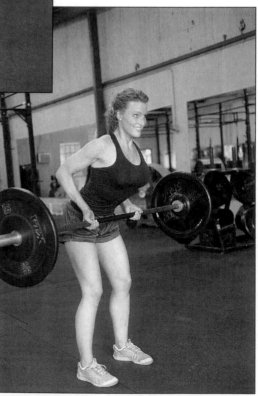

Back   **Pull-ups**

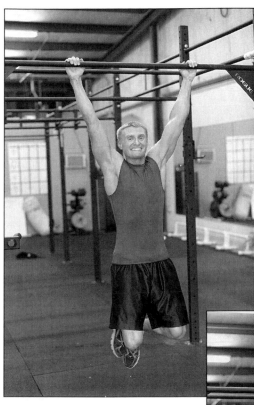

Pull-ups - Start

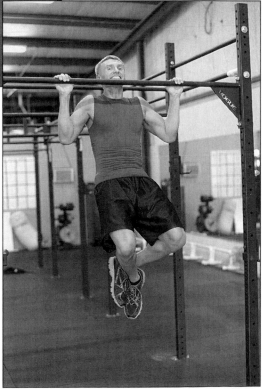

Pull-ups - Finish

Back

Assisted Pull-ups

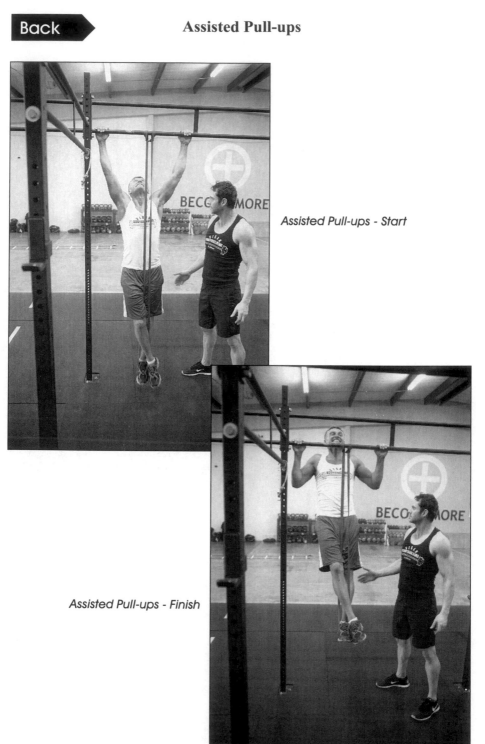

Assisted Pull-ups - Start

Assisted Pull-ups - Finish

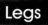 **Legs**

Walking Weighted Lunges

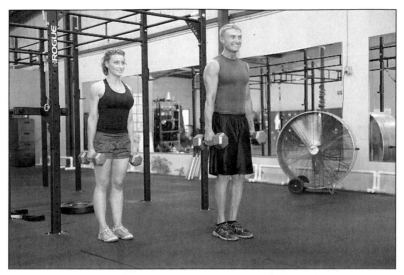

Dumbbell Walking Lunges - Start

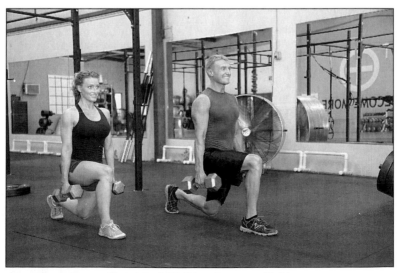

Dumbbell Walking Lunges - Finish

Legs ▶

Bodyweight Squats

Bodyweight Squats - Start

Bodyweight Squats - Finish

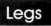 **Legs**

One-legged Squats

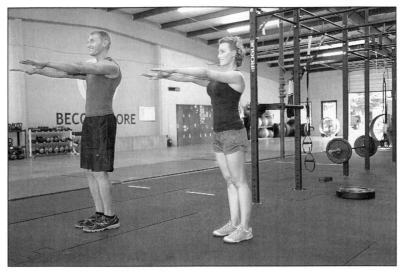

One Legged Squats - Start

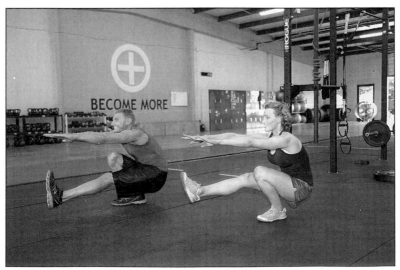

One Legged Squats - Finish

Standing Weighted Calf Raises

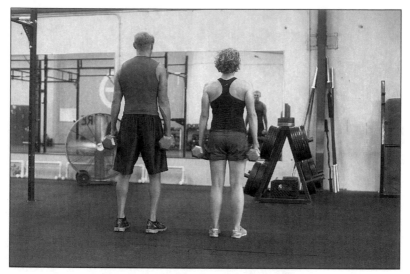

Standing Dumbbell Calf Raises - Start

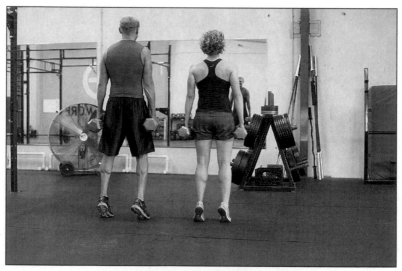

Standing Dumbbell Calf Raises - Finish

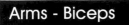

Arms - Biceps

Hammer Curls

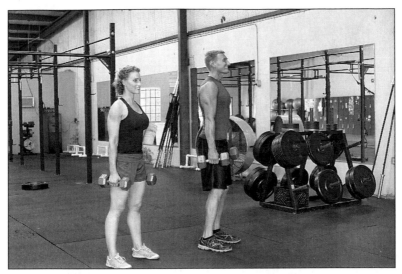

Dumbbell Hammer Curls - Start

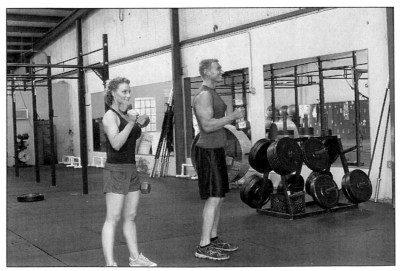

Dumbbell Hammer Curls - Finish

Arms - Biceps ▶ **Concentration Curls**

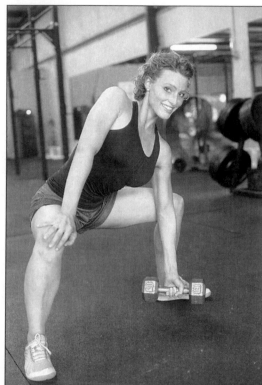

Concentration Curls - Start

Concentration Curls - Finish

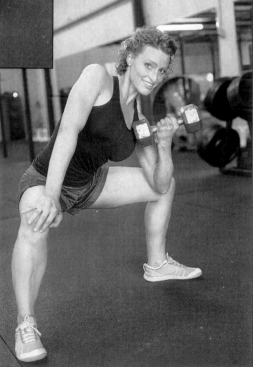

Arms - Triceps   ## Skull Crushers

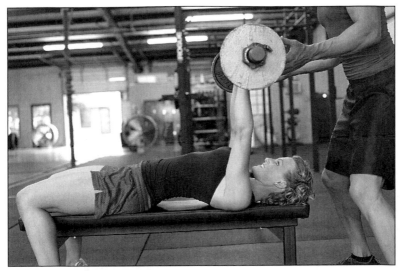

Skull Crushers - Start

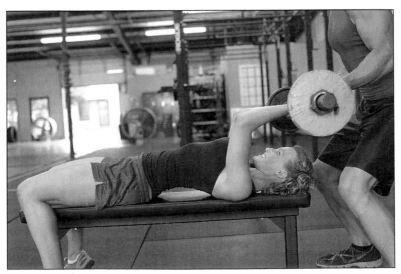

Skull Crushers - Finish

Arms - Triceps ▶ **Narrow-grip Bench Press**

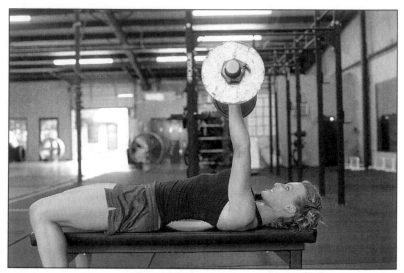

Narrow-grip Bench Press - Start

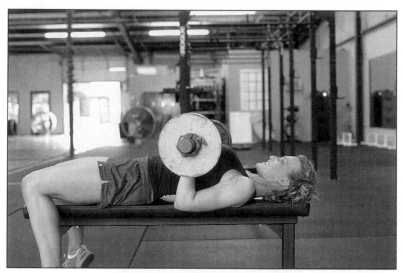

Narrow-grip Bench Press - Finish

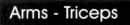 **Arms - Triceps** **Dumbbell Kickbacks**

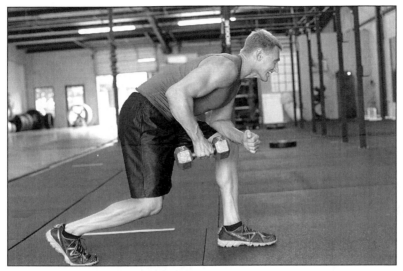

Dumbbell Kickbacks - Start

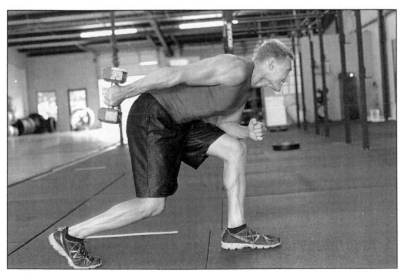

Dumbbell Kickbacks - Finish

Hanging Leg Raises

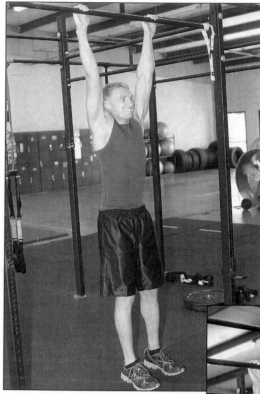

Hanging Leg Raises - Start

Hanging Leg Raises - Finish

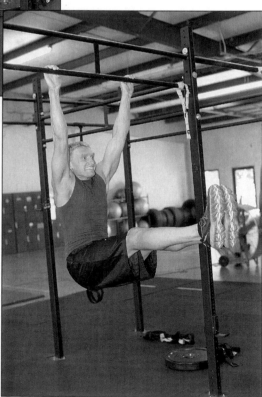

Plank

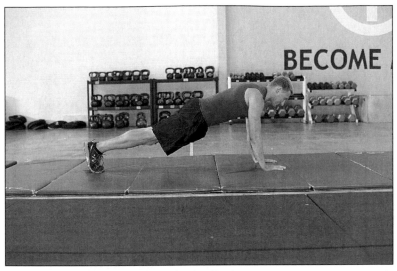

Plank - Start

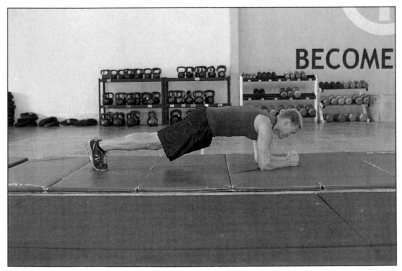

Plank - Finish

Pike on Yoga Ball

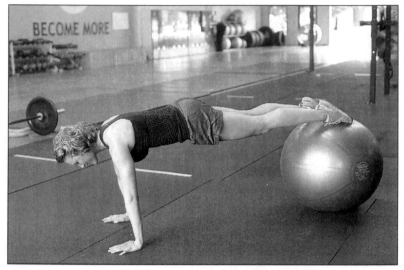

Pike on Yoga Ball - Start

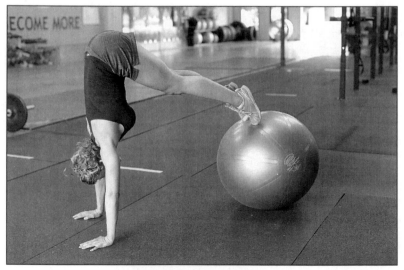

Pike on Yoga Ball - Finish

Partner Sit-ups

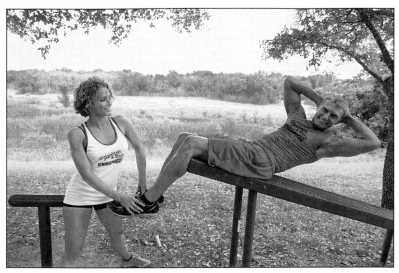

Partner Sit-ups - Start

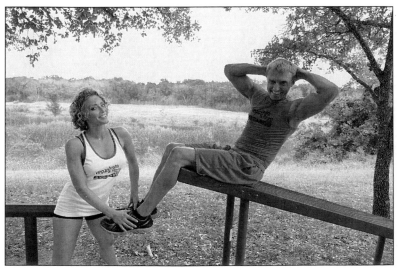

Partner Sit-ups - Finish

Partner Medicine Ball Crunches

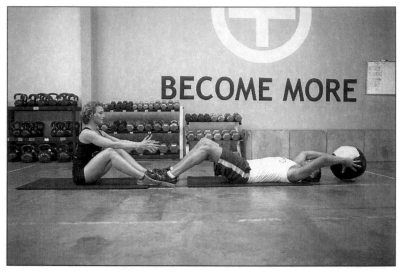

Partner Medicine Ball Sit-ups - Start

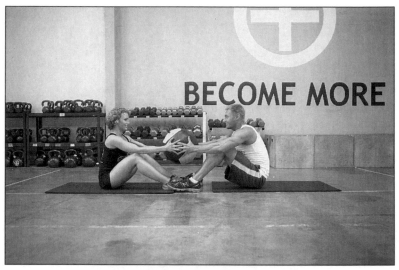

Partner Medicine Ball Sit-ups - Finish

Total Body Workouts

Not everyone has access to a gym to use the types of equipment that is outlined above, or have that kind of equipment at home. If you do not have access to a gym, or you prefer not to go to one, and don't have weight training equipment at home, bodyweight exercises and total body workouts just might be your best approach.

If you don't have access to the equipment to do the exercises that Mindy and I demonstrate in the photos above, you can get a tremendous workout by using just your body, to do common exercises such as push-ups, squats, lunges, jumps, sprints, and so many more. You can pick any one of those exercises and train to exhaustion in a pretty short amount of time, mere seconds or minutes, depending on the exercise. You can alter your pace, depth, repetition range, and level of intensity to change the dynamic and impact of each exercise. I lead group fitness classes at various health conferences without any equipment at all, just using our own bodies, and nearly everyone, regardless of their level of fitness, is exhausted by the end. That is because no matter what the exercise is, you can always perform repetitions to failure and you can use drop sets and super sets to lead to exhaustion with movements as simple as bodyweight push-ups, squats, lunges, static holds, and jumps.

If total body exercises are more in line with your interest, consider some of the following total body workouts to incorporate into your exercise schedule.

Total Body Workout Sample #1 ▶ Upper Body Exercises

Warm-up (10-15 minutes)

Perform the following in a continuous motion for at least 10 minutes with 30 second intervals performing each exercise, followed by 30 seconds of jogging in place between each exercise:

- Arm circles for 1 minute forward and 1 minute backward
- Jog in place for 1 minute and swing your arms in and out and side to side to loosen up
- Jog in place for 30 seconds
- High knees for 30 seconds
- Jog in place for 30 seconds
- Heels to glutes for 30 seconds

- Jog in place for 30 seconds
- Jumping Jacks/Jills for 30 seconds
- Jog in place for 30 seconds
- High skips for 30 seconds
- Jog in place for 30 seconds
- Squats for 30 seconds
- Jog in place for 30 seconds
- Push-ups for 30 seconds
- Jog in place for 30 seconds
- Invisible jump rope for 30 seconds
- Jog in place for 30 seconds
- Star jumps for 30 seconds
- Jog in place for 30 seconds
- Jog in place for 1 minute and swing your arms in and out and side to side

Stretching (5-10 minutes)

Stretch your quads, hamstrings, calves, abdominals, arms, chest, shoulders, and back through a variety of basic stretches to loosen up after the warm-up. Stretching is not to be overlooked and should be performed once some form of preliminary exercise has been completed to increase circulation, improve flexibility, and warm-up joints and muscles that will be used in the forthcoming exercises.

Upper body exercises (20-30 minutes or as long as you want)

Push-ups x as many reps as you can for 3-5 sets

Plank x as long as you can hold it for 3-5 sets

Push-up jacks x as many as you can for 3-5 sets

Slow moving Spiderman push-ups x as many as you can do for 3-5 sets

Cool Down/Stretching (5-10 minutes)

Arm circles for 1 minute forward and 1 minute backward

Jog in place for 2 minutes

Stretch your quads, hamstrings, calves, abdominals, arms, chest, shoulders, and back through a variety of basic stretches to stretch muscles out after the workout.

Total Body Workout Sample #2 — Lower Body Exercises

Warm-up (10-15 minutes)

Perform the following in a continuous motion for at least 10 minutes with 30 second intervals performing each exercise, followed by 30 seconds of jogging in place between each exercise:

- Ankle circles for 30 seconds forward, 30 seconds backward with each foot
- Arm circles for 1 minute forward and 1 minute backward
- Jog in place for 1 minute and swing your arms in and out and side to side to loosen up
- Jog in place for 30 seconds
- High knees for 30 seconds
- Jog in place for 30 seconds
- Heels to glutes for 30 seconds
- Jog in place for 30 seconds
- Jumping Jacks/Jills for 30 seconds
- Jog in place for 30 seconds
- High skips for 30 seconds
- Jog in place for 30 seconds
- Squats for 30 seconds
- Jog in place for 30 seconds
- Lunges for 30 seconds
- Jog in place for 30 seconds

- Invisible jump rope for 30 seconds
- Jog in place for 30 seconds
- Star jumps for 30 seconds
- Jog in place for 30 seconds
- Speed skaters for 30 seconds
- Jog in place for 1 minute and swing your arms in and out and side to side

Stretching (5-10 minutes)

Stretch your quads, hamstrings, calves, abdominals, arms, chest, shoulders, and back through a variety of basic stretches to loosen up after the warm-up. Stretching is not to be overlooked and should be performed once some form of preliminary exercise has been performed to increase circulation, improve flexibility and warm-up joints and muscles that will be used in the forthcoming exercises.

Lower body exercises (20-30 minutes or as long as you want)

Squats x as many reps as you can for 3-5 sets

Lunges x as many reps as you can for 3-5 sets

Star jumps x as many reps as you can for 3-5 sets

Wall sits for as long as you can x 3-5 sets

Cool Down/Stretching (5-10 minutes)

Ankle circles for 30 seconds forward, 30 seconds backward with each foot

Arm circles for 1 minute forward and 1 minute backward

Jog in place for 2 minutes

Stretch your quads, hamstrings, calves, abdominals, arms, chest, shoulders, and back through a variety of basic stretches to stretch muscles out after the workout.

Total Body Workout Sample #3   **Total Body Exercises**

Warm-up (10-15 minutes)

Perform the following in a continuous motion for at least 10 minutes with 30 second intervals performing each exercise, followed by 30 seconds of jogging in place between each exercise:

- Ankle circles for 30 seconds forward, 30 seconds backward with each foot
- Arm circles for 1 minute forward and 1 minute backward
- Jog in place for 1 minute and swing your arms in and out and side to side to loosen up
- Jog in place for 30 seconds
- High knees for 30 seconds
- Jog in place for 30 seconds
- Heels to glutes for 30 seconds
- Jog in place for 30 seconds
- Jumping Jacks/Jills for 30 seconds
- Jog in place for 30 seconds
- High skips for 30 seconds
- Jog in place for 30 seconds
- Squats for 30 seconds
- Jog in place for 30 seconds
- Lunges for 30 seconds
- Jog in place for 30 seconds
- Invisible jump rope for 30 seconds
- Jog in place for 30 seconds
- Star jumps for 30 seconds
- Jog in place for 30 seconds
- Speed skaters for 30 seconds
- Jog in place for 1 minute and swing your arms in and out and side to side

Stretching (5-10 minutes)

Stretch your quads, hamstrings, calves, abdominals, arms, chest, shoulders, and back through a variety of basic stretches to loosen up after the warm-up. Stretching is not to be overlooked and should be performed once some form of preliminary exercise has been performed to increase circulation, improve flexibility and warm-up joints and muscles that will be used in the forthcoming exercises.

Total Body Exercises (20-30 minutes or as long as you want)

Mountain climbers x as many as possible for 3-5 sets

Burpees x as many as possible for 3-5 sets

Star jumps x as many as possible for 3-5 sets

Jump squat + push-up combo x as many as possible x 3-5 sets

Cool Down/Stretching (5-10 minutes)

Ankle circles for 30 seconds forward, 30 seconds backward with each foot

Arm circles for 1 minute forward and 1 minute backward

Jog in place for 2 minutes

Stretch your quads, hamstrings, calves, abdominals, arms, chest, shoulders, and back through a variety of basic stretches to stretch muscles out after the workout.

Total Body Exercises ▶ **Box Jumps**

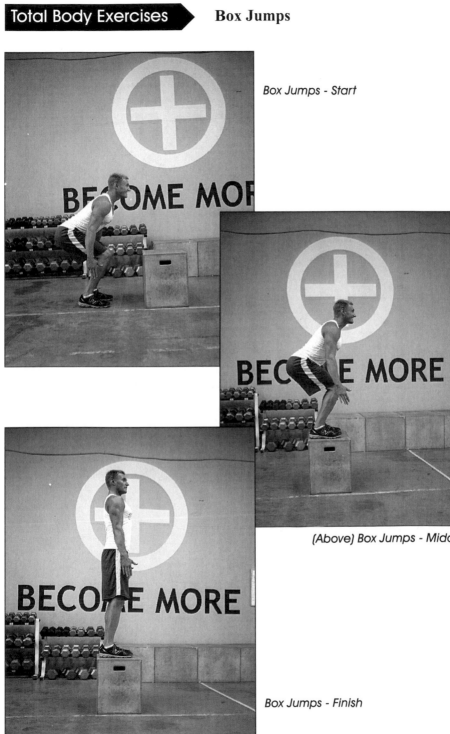

Box Jumps - Start

(Above) Box Jumps - Middle

Box Jumps - Finish

Stretching and Recovery

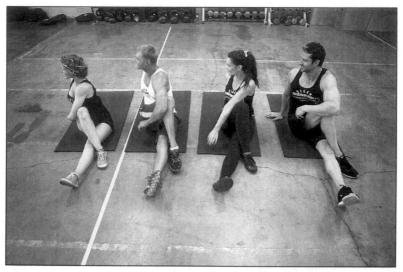

Seated twisting lower back stretch

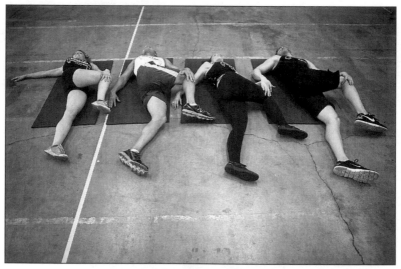

Lying twisting lower back stretch

Stretching and Recovery

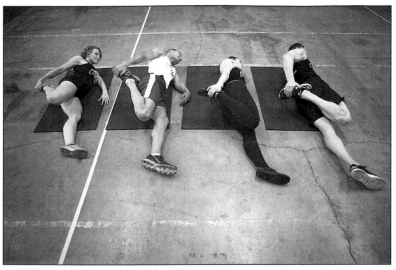

Lying quadriceps stretch

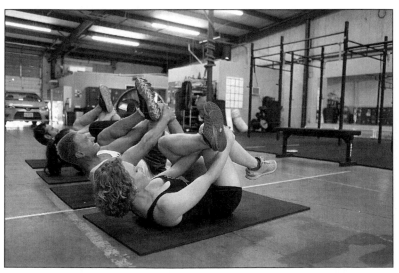

Lying glute stretch

Shred It!

Stretching and Recovery

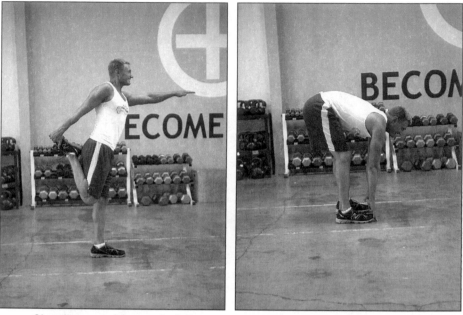

Standing quadriceps stretch   *Standing hamstring stretch*

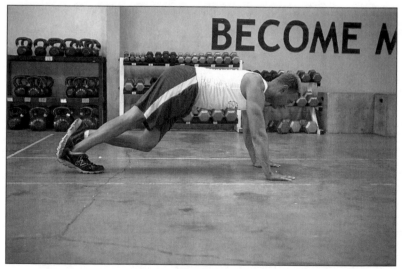

Calf stretch

Foam Roller

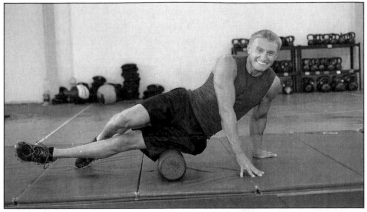

Foam Roller - IT Band

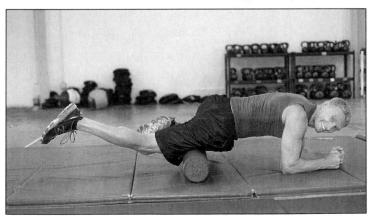

Foam Roller - Quadriceps

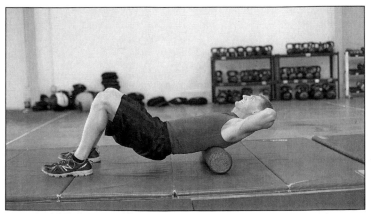

Foam Roller - Errectors

Recap

You all have your own unique goals to change your current level of health and fitness into something that you desire and strive for. Some of you will build muscle and others will get more shredded than you've ever been by leaning out as a result of your tailor-made approach to burning fat. Whatever you aim to accomplish, I am confident the exercise programs listed above will help you get there. Regardless of the style of training you decide to pursue, make an effort to document it in a training journal, whether a physical one as mentioned previously, or online. I have training and nutrition journals available on my website, www.veganbodybuilding.com, to help you stay consistent and accountable to follow through with your goals. They are designed to keep you motivated and inspired with their unique approach including images, tips, quotes, and featured athletes, among the actual journal pages to record your workouts and meals.

Feel free to join our online plant-based athlete communities as well. We have numerous resources for you to record your training and nutrition journals online where you can get feedback and input from others, and it is a prime environment for transparency to keep you moving forward. Links to all of our online forums are on www.veganbodybuilding.com.

Now that you are equipped with a plethora of helpful exercises, including demonstrations of many, it's time to fuel your body and replenish, repair and rebuild through sound nutrition. The following recipes from numerous cookbook authors, chefs and athletes will provide you with the other part of the equation. Exercise is only half the battle, what you decide to eat will determine your overall health outcome. Wishing you all the best. Enjoy everything the plant-based kitchen has to offer.

Primary exercise photos by Austin Barbisch
Additional exercise photos by Sarah Brightly and Brenda Carey

– CHAPTER 10 –

Recipes

In this chapter I will reveal to you precisely how unskilled I am in the kitchen, but will show you how I am still able to be successful, eat creatively, and support my fitness goals. Perhaps the three total recipes in my 317-page book, *Vegan Bodybuilding & Fitness*, was an indication that I'm not exactly Betty Crocker or Julia Child. I build my own meal plans, but I am not an avid follower of recipes.

I have a number of colleagues whom I respect and hold in very high regard that have contributed some outstanding recipes to help you achieve your health and fitness goals. I recruited chefs, cookbook authors, and fellow plant-based athletes to contribute awesome recipes for this chapter. I invite you to try the wonderful culinary creations our Vegan Bodybuilding & Fitness team members have produced for you to enjoy.

Marcella Torres
Plant-based author, athlete and business owner
VeganMuscleandFitness.com

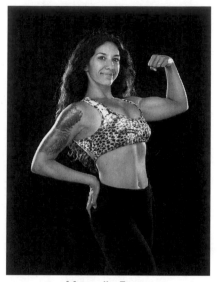

Marcella Torres
Photo by Melissa Schwartz - theveganrevolution.net

Marcella, formerly a professional mathematician, is now a competitive vegan bodybuilder, professional dancer, coauthor of *The Vegan Muscle & Fitness Guide to Bodybuilding Competitions*, coauthor of the Vegan Muscle & Fitness blog, and co-owner of plant-based personal training studio Root Force Personal Training in Richmond, VA with husband Derek Tresize.

While a whole-foods, plant-based diet based on a variety of legumes, vegetables, fruits, whole grains, and a small amount of nuts and seeds is always going to be optimal for both muscle gain and fat loss, you may want to adjust your menu at times to focus on a particular goal. For example, when Derek and I are in the gaining phase of our bodybuilding competition prep, we eat more calories, but when we're striving to lose fat in the weeks before a contest the focus of our menu becomes nutrient-dense foods rather than calorie-dense foods. However, our diet at all times is based on the same whole-plant foods. I want to share an example with you of how I keep my meal planning straightforward by simply adjusting my staple recipes. The beauty of a plant-based menu is that there is no gaping divide between a fat loss diet and a muscle gain diet, and that achieving either goal becomes straightforward when all of your options are healthy.

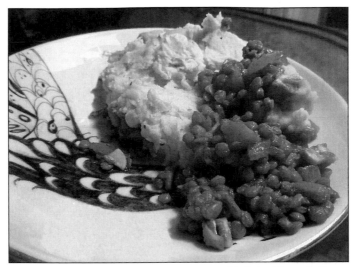

Photo by Marcella Torres

Lentil Shepherd's Pie

The lentil filling is the same in either version of this recipe—only the topping varies. For the lower calorie version, choose the Cauliflower Topping and for the richer high-calorie version, choose the Mashed Potato Topping. This makes a great potluck dish!

- 1 cup cooked lentils, optionally cooked in vegetable broth
- 1 tbsp ketchup
- 1 tbsp low sodium soy sauce
- 1 tsp vegan Worcestershire sauce, optional
- 1 tsp thyme
- 1/4 tsp marjoram
- 1/4 tsp paprika
- 1/4 tsp onion powder
- pepper to taste

Mix all ingredients in a mixing bowl. Preheat oven to 350° while you prepare one of the following toppings. When the topping is complete, assemble the pie: place filling in a medium-sized ovenproof casserole dish and smooth topping over it. Broil until the top is lightly browned. Oven temperatures on broil vary quite a bit, so you will need to keep an eye on it!

Cauliflower Topping

> 1 cauliflower
>
> Non-dairy milk
>
> Salt and pepper to taste

Set a large pot of water to boil. Cut the cauliflower into large florets and add to the boiling water. Boil for 15 minutes or until the cauliflower is tender and easily pierced with a fork. Drain and add to a large bowl. Mash with a potato masher, adding non-dairy milk as necessary—but not too much! Season with salt and pepper. Alternatively, you can process the cauliflower in a food processor. Proceed with lentil shepherd's pie recipe.

Mashed Potato Topping

> 1/3 cup cashews, soaked in water overnight*
>
> 5 medium russet potatoes, peeled and diced
>
> salt and pepper to taste

*Soaking overnight is unnecessary if you have a Vitamix or other powerful blender. Add cashews to blender and just cover with cold water. Blend at high speed until very smooth; this will likely take a few minutes. Set aside. Add potatoes to a large pot, cover with water, and bring to a boil. Cook until potatoes can be easily pierced with a fork—about 10-15 minutes. Drain. In a large bowl, mash the potatoes with the blended cashews and salt and pepper to taste until smooth. Proceed with lentil shepherd's pie recipe.

Arvid Beck
Competitive bodybuilder
Arvidbeck.de

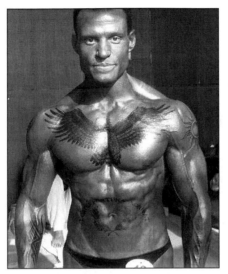

Arvid Beck

Arvid is a competitive bodybuilder from Germany. His current diet is based on whole foods, with an emphasis on carbohydrates (up to 80 percent) and little fat (usually around 10 percent), and doesn't include any protein powders. His staples are grains, legumes, vegetables, and fruits.

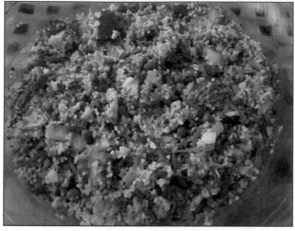

Photo by Arvid Beck

Hot Couscous Salad

250 grams couscous

250 grams tomatoes

300 grams carrots

1 can peas (280 grams in cooked state)

5 ounces freshly pressed lemon juice (3 lemons)

1 onion

1/2 bunch parsley

2 tbsp sambal oelek

Mixed pepper

(Salt)

Put the couscous into a huge bowl and pour about 20 ounces of boiling water in there. Let the couscous steep for at least 10 minutes, until all the water is soaked up.

In the meantime you can press the lemon juice and prepare the vegetables. Cut the onion and the tomatoes into little pieces, and chop the parsley with a knife or any other kitchen utensil. Use a rasp to cut the carrots into little strips.

When the couscous is ready, sprinkle (plenty of) pepper over it (and a bit of salt if desired), add the lemon juice and two tablespoonful of sambal oelek. Stir properly until the spices are evenly spread. After that add the vegetables and peas and stir again. Finished!

This salad will give you a lot of carbohydrates, protein, fiber, vitamins and minerals. The amount should be enough for at least three servings.

Nutritional Value

Calories:	1316 calories
Carbohydrates:	235.8 grams
Fiber:	42.7 grams
Protein:	53.9 grams
Fat:	7.8 grams

Tess Challis
Author, vegan chef, cooking instructor, and wellness coach
Radianthealth-innerweath.com

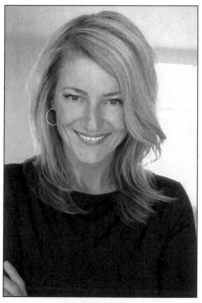

Tess Challis
Photo by Melissa Schwartz -
theveganrevolution.net

Tess began her holistic health journey in her late teens. After numerous health ailments (severe acne, obesity, strep throat, constant illnesses, anxiety, and depression), she found that a healthy vegan diet along with an inner wellness regime of meditation, affirmations, and visualization made a world of difference.

Tess's books include *Radiant Health, Inner Wealth, The Two-Week Wellness Solution, Radiance 4 Life,* and *Get Waisted: 100 Addictively Delicious Plant-Based Entrées.* Tess lives in Florida.

Key for Tess's recipes:

GF = Gluten-free   SF = Sugar-free   R = Raw

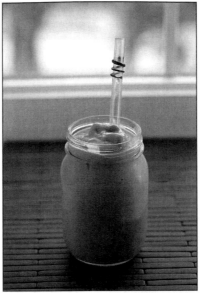

Photo by Janet Malowany

3 Ingredient Strawberry Milkshake

You'll be surprised how creamy, sweet, and delicious this simple shake is. This one, incidentally, is my daughter's favorite—she asks for it almost every day!

> 3/4 cup raw cashews
>
> 1 cup chopped frozen bananas (from very ripe bananas)
>
> 2/3 cups frozen strawberries

Blend well (preferably in a high-speed blender), adding 2/3 cup water (just enough to blend) until the mixture is smooth and creamy. Serve immediately.

NOTE: If you do not have a high-speed blender (Vitamix or Blendtec), you will need to soak the cashews in water for a few hours before blending.

GF/SF/Green (according to the guidelines in Tess's books)

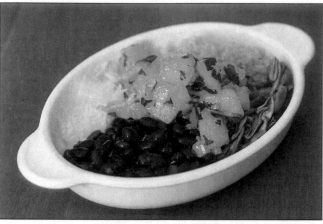

Photo by Janet Malowany

Black Bean and Rice Bowl with Mango Salsa

Recipe from *Get Waisted: 100 Addictively Delicious
Plant-Based Entrées* (by Tess Challis and Dr. Mary Clifton)

The abundance of flavorful, fresh salsa brings all the other ingredients to life!

Mango Salsa

2 cups diced mango (the flesh of about 2 large mangoes)

1/4 cup **each**: finely minced white onion and chopped cilantro

2 tbsps fresh lime juice

1/4 tsp **each**: sea salt and dried chili (red pepper) flakes

Salad

2 cups cooked brown rice

1 1/2 cups cooked black beans (one can of black beans, drained and rinsed)

3/4 cup **each**: grated carrots and chopped or grated red cabbage

1) Make the mango salsa: Toss all of the salsa ingredients together in a medium bowl until well combined and overly enticing. Set aside.

2) Layer the salad ingredients in a bowl. Top with the salsa and serve. Enjoy your colorful, health-promoting fiesta in a bowl!

GF/SF/Green (according to the guidelines in Tess's books)

Ginger Lime Carrot Soup

Recipe from
Radiance 4 Life
(foreword by
Robert Cheeke)

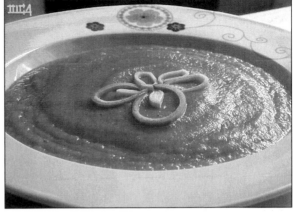

Photo by Olga Vasijeva

This soup is pure, vibrant, delicious health in a bowl! If it were any healthier, it might be illegal in certain states. In fact, let's just keep this between you and me.

> One medium sweet potato, baked until soft (1 cup sweet potato flesh)
>
> 3 medium-large carrots, trimmed and chopped (1 1/2 cups chopped carrots)*
>
> 3 cups almond milk (plain and unsweetened)
>
> 2 tbsps grated fresh ginger
>
> 1 tbsp fresh lime juice
>
> 2 large cloves garlic, minced or pressed
>
> 1 1/4 tsp sea salt
>
> 1/4 - 1/2 tsp ground cayenne (1/2 tsp will make it very spicy)
>
> **For serving:** 1/4 cup chopped cilantro

1) Bake the sweet potato if you haven't already done so. Remove the skin and set aside.

2) Place the sweet potato in a high-speed blender (a Vitamix or Blendtec) along with the remaining ingredients (except the cilantro). Blend well, until velvety smooth.

Serve immediately, topped with cilantro.

GF/SF/Green (according to the guidelines in Tess's books)

*NOTE: If you don't have a high-speed blender, you'll need to roast the carrots along with the potato so that they will blend up smoothly.

Raw Cinnamon Rolls

Recipe from
Radiance 4 Life
(foreword by Robert Cheeke)

Think of these as a quick, delicious, healthy alternative to packaged energy bars. Since they're so nutrient-dense, just one little roll can be surprisingly satisfying.

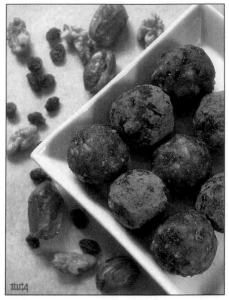

Photo by Olga Vasijeva

P.S. I like to also call these "RC Rolls" since Robert (Cheeke) likes them so much! They really are the perfect treat for on-the-go energy snacking.

> 1 cup raw walnuts
>
> 1/2 cup raisins
>
> 1/2 cup (packed) pitted dates (about 12 dates)
>
> 1 tbsp cinnamon
>
> 1/4 tsp **each**: sea salt and ground nutmeg

1) Place all of the ingredients in a food processor. Blend until well combined and very crumbly, but don't over blend—you want to retain some texture.

2) Pull out small pieces of the mixture and roll into 1-inch balls with your hands. These will store in an airtight container, refrigerated, for several weeks or more.

Makes 18 rolls (9 servings)

GF/SF/Green (according to the guidelines in Tess's books)

Thai Red Curry Noodles

Recipe from *Get Waisted: 100 Addictively Delicious Plant-Based Entrées* (by Tess Challis and Dr. Mary Clifton)

These flavorful, saucy noodles boast loads of antioxidants—plus, they come together in under 30 minutes! Perfection happens, and when it does I like to sit back, laugh, and eat red curry noodles.

> 8 oz. whole grain rice noodles, the kind you would use for Pad Thai (I use Annie Chun's brown rice noodles)
>
> 2 tbsps Thai red curry paste (such as Thai Kitchen brand)
>
> One 14 oz. can low-fat coconut milk
>
> 5 large cloves garlic, minced or pressed
>
> 2 tbsps grated fresh ginger
>
> 1/2 cup (packed) **each**: finely chopped green onions and chopped cilantro
>
> 1/4 cup fresh lime juice
>
> 1/4 cup (packed) fresh basil, cut into thin ribbons
>
> 1 tsp sea salt

1) Prepare the noodles according to the directions on their package.

2) While the noodles are cooking, you can get the rest of the dish together. In a large bowl, place the curry paste and a little of the coconut milk. Whisk together until smooth. Add the remaining coconut milk and whisk again until emulsified.

3) Add the remaining ingredients to the bowl and stir well.

4) Once the noodles are al dente, drain them very well and add them to the bowl. Stir gently to thoroughly combine. Serve at room temperature.

GF/SF/Green (according to the guidelines in Tess's books)

Classic
Mixed Bean Salad

Recipe from
Get Waisted:
100 Addictively
Delicious Plant-Based
Entrées (by Tess Challis
and Dr. Mary Clifton)

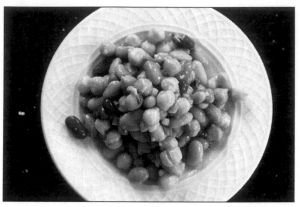

Photo by Janet Malowany

This fat-free "salad" is perfect as a main dish for summer potlucks, light dinners, and can even be served over spinach or greens.

> One 15 oz. can garbanzo beans (chickpeas)
>
> One 15 oz. can mixed beans (a blend of kidney beans, pinto beans, and black beans)
>
> 1 cup thawed, shelled edamame
>
> 3/4 cup minced scallions (green onions)
>
> 1/4 cup apple cider vinegar
>
> 2 tbsps each: agave nectar and fresh lime juice
>
> 1 tsp ground (dried) yellow mustard powder
>
> 3/4 tsp sea salt (or less if you prefer)

1) Place the garbanzo beans, mixed beans, and edamame in a strainer (over a sink) and rinse well with water. Let drain while you're tossing the remaining items together.

2) Place all of the remaining ingredients in a medium-large bowl and stir well to combine.

3) Add the drained beans and edamame to the bowl and gently toss well so that all of the ingredients are thoroughly combined. Voila! Bean happiness at your fingertips. This dish will stay fresh for up to a week when refrigerated in an airtight container.

GF/SF/Green (according to the guidelines in Tess's books)

Indian Spiced
Super Grain Cereal

Recipe from *Radiant Health, Inner Wealth*

Here is a fabulously healthy way to start the day when you **really** need some nourishment!

- 1/4 cup each: dry amaranth **and** dry quinoa, washed well and drained
- 1 cup water
- 5 whole cardamom pods (preferably green)
- 1/8 tsp ground ginger
- 1/2 tsp ground cinnamon
- 1/4 tsp vanilla extract
- 1/4 cup nondairy milk
- 1 tbsp pure maple syrup

Optional

- 2 tbsps raisins (or pitted, chopped dried dates)

1) In a small pan, bring the amaranth, quinoa, water, cardamom, ginger, cinnamon, and vanilla to a boil over high heat, stirring well.

2) Reduce heat to low and simmer for about 10 minutes, or until the grains are tender and the liquid is absorbed.

3) Remove the cardamom pods and add the remaining ingredients. Stir well and serve.

30 minutes or under

GF/SF/Green (according to the guidelines in Tess's books)

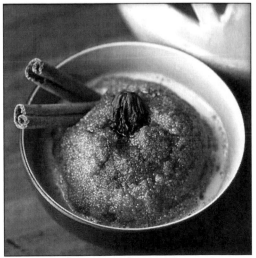

Photo by Michelle Bebber

Southwest Spring Rolls with Green Chili Sauce

Recipe from *Radiant Health, Inner Wealth*

This idea came to me when I was trying to create a fresh spring roll that would also double as a satisfying lunch. Although pairing southwest fillings with an Asian concept is a little "out there," so am I.

Green Chili Sauce

> 1 tbsp brown rice flour
>
> 1 1/2 cups roasted, peeled, finely chopped green chilies, thawed if frozen
>
> 1 tbsp coconut sugar
>
> 1/4 cup plus 1 tsp **fresh** lime juice
>
> 1 - 1 1/4 tsp sea salt
>
> 5 medium cloves garlic, minced or pressed

Fillings

> 1/3 cup pine nuts (toasted in a dry pan until lightly browned)
>
> 1 ripe avocado, peeled, pitted, and chopped
>
> 1/2 cup grated (or julienne cut) carrot
>
> 1/2 cup (packed) chopped fresh cilantro
>
> 4 scallions (green onions), trimmed and cut into eight 3-inch spears

Talkin' Sheet

> 8 spring roll skins/rice paper sheets (preferably brown rice wraps if available)

1) *First, make the sauce:* Place the rice flour, chilies, and coconut sugar in a medium saucepan and whisk well until thoroughly combined. Cook over medium-high heat for about five minutes, stirring often, until a bit thicker in consistency. Turn off the heat and stir in the lime juice, sea salt, and garlic. Combine well and set aside.

2) Prepare the other fillings and set them aside.

3) Find a pan or bowl large enough to put the rice paper wrappers in. Fill it two inches high with lukewarm or cool water. Place a sheet of rice paper in the water, making sure it's covered entirely with the water. In less than a minute it will be soft. Don't over-soak the wrapper, as it will tear more easily if you do.

4) Remove the wrapper and allow any excess water to drip off of it. Lay it flat on a clean surface. Place a little of each filling item in the middle of the wrapper. You'll want to use too much filling if you're like me, but try and restrain yourself. The wraps will roll up much more neatly and stay enclosed if you don't overfill them. This takes practice, friends—but you can master it.

5) Roll the bottom of the rice paper wrapper up and over the fillings. Next, fold the left and right sides over the filling. If you can maintain parallel lines, it will produce a more even looking wrap. Finally, finish rolling it all of the way up. The rice paper will self-seal, so just set the spring roll aside and repeat this process until all of your fillings are used up. Serve with the sauce and enjoy!

Makes 8 spring rolls

GF/SF/Green (according to the guidelines in Tess's books)

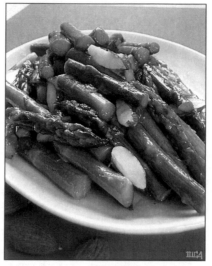

Photo by Olga Vasijeva

Apricot Glazed Asparagus

Recipe from *The Two-Week Wellness Solution*

What a delicious way to get in your veggies!

> 2 cups chopped asparagus (trimmed and cut into 1-inch pieces)
> 1 1/2 tsp **each**: water and tamari
> 2 tbsps apricot fruit spread (all-fruit jam)
> 1 medium clove garlic, minced or pressed

Optional

> 1 tsp slivered or sliced almonds, toasted (dry toast in a pan over medium heat until lightly browned and aromatic)

1) In a medium skillet set to medium-high heat, sauté the asparagus in the water and tamari, stirring often. When the asparagus turns bright green and is crisp-tender, remove from heat. This should take well under 5 minutes.

2) Gently stir the apricot fruit spread and garlic into the asparagus until well mixed. Serve plain or topped with the almonds.

30 minutes or under

GF/Green (according to the guidelines in Tess's books)

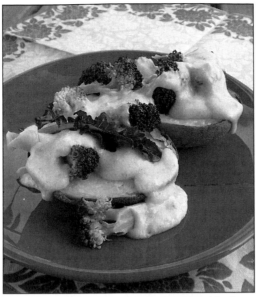

Photo by Olga Vasijeva

Cheesy Broccoli Baked Potato

Recipe from *Get Waisted: 100 Addictively Delicious Plant-Based Entrées* (by Tess Challis and Dr. Mary Clifton)

Baked potatoes as an entrée? Why yes! Potatoes have unfairly gotten a bad rap in the weight loss arena, but in reality there are few more perfect foods. Potatoes are filling, fiber-rich, extremely high in potassium, fat-free, and full of vitamins and minerals. If you keep the cheesy mix on hand, this will become a favorite easy go-to meal—at least that's what plays out in our house!

Ingredients

    4 large potatoes, scrubbed (skins on)

    6 cups broccoli, cut into bite-size pieces

Cheesy Mix

    1 cup raw cashews

    1 1/4 cups nutritional yeast

    1/2 cup rolled oats

    1/4 cup arrowroot

2 tbsps each: seasoned salt and garlic granules (granulated garlic)

1 1/2 tbsp onion granules (granulated onion)

1/2 tsp ground turmeric

1) Preheat your oven to 400 F. Place the potatoes in the oven (just right onto the racks is fine). Bake for about 45 minutes, or until tender.

2) While the potatoes are baking, you can assemble the rest of your dish. First, place all of the ingredients for the cheesy mix in a food processor. Blend until a fine powder. This cheesy mix will store in the fridge (in an airtight container) for months—although it never lasts that long in our house! Set it aside.

3) When the potatoes are almost tender, steam the broccoli until tender and bright green. Set aside.

4) Place 1 cup of cheesy mix with 2 cups water in a small pot, set to medium heat (it is a 2:1 ratio, water to mix). Whisking often, cook until thickened. This will take well under 5 minutes.

5) To assemble: Place the baked potatoes on plates, cut them open, and mash them. Top with some broccoli and pour a generous serving of the sauce on top. Enjoy!

GF/SF/Green (according to the guidelines in Tess's books)

-

Rawcho Cheese Dip

Recipe from *Radiance 4 Life*

This dip will convince you, once and for all, that healthy food can taste amazing.

1/2 cup raw cashews

4 oz. jar pimientos, drained

1/4 cup nutritional yeast powder

3 tbsps fresh lemon juice

3 medium-large cloves garlic, peeled

2 tbsps water

1 tsp granulated onion

3/4 tsp sea salt

1/4 tsp ground cayenne

Blend all of the ingredients in a food processor (or high speed blender such as a Blendtec or Vitamix) until completely smooth. Serve cold or at room temperature with raw vegetables, baked tortilla chips, or raw crackers. This will store, refrigerated in an airtight container, for at least a week.

Makes about 1 cup of dip (4 servings)

GF/SF/Blue (according to the guidelines in Tess's books)

Green Velvet Guacamole

Recipe from *Radiance 4 Life*

Here's a lower fat, full-flavor guacamole that will rock your socks. Serve as a topping for anything and everything Mexican.

Flesh of 2 medium avocados

1 cup shelled edamame (thawed if frozen)

5 tbsps fresh lime juice

3 large cloves garlic, peeled

1 tsp sea salt

In a food processor or blender, emulsify all of the ingredients until silky smooth.

This will store, refrigerated in an airtight container, for several days.

Makes 8-10 servings

30 minutes or under

GF/Green/R (according to the guidelines in Tess's books)

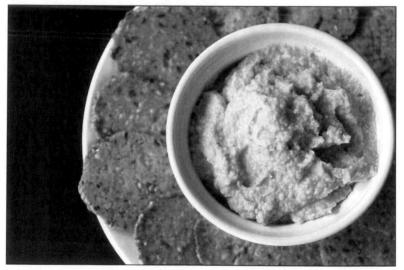

Photo by Janet Malowany

Moroccan Barley-Spinach Toss

Recipe from *Radiant Health, Inner Wealth*

I'm a big fan of Moroccan seasonings—sweet, tart, and savory all at once. Yum!

> 1 cup dry barley, soaked in water overnight, drained, then allowed to sit for several hours, or until softened

Sweet-Savory Sauce

> 1 tsp **each**: ground cumin and minced organic orange zest
>
> 3/4 cup fresh squeezed orange juice
>
> 4 tsps **each**: fresh lemon juice and very finely minced onion
>
> 2 tsps ground cinnamon
>
> 2 tbsps raw agave nectar

Simple Salad

> 1/2 cup raisins
>
> 1 cup (packed) baby spinach, cut into very thin ribbons or minced
>
> Fresh mint, minced (about 1 1/2 tbsps)

1) Stir the sauce ingredients together in a medium sized bowl until well combined.

2) Add the sprouted barley, raisins, and spinach to the sauce and toss to thoroughly combine.

3) Allow the mixture to marinate for at least 20 minutes, stirring occasionally to saturate the sauce into everything. If you do have the time to marinate this for an hour, that's even better. After the dish has finished marinating, add the mint and serve.

GF/SF/Green (according to the guidelines in Tess's books)

Mexican Polenta Bowl

Recipe from *Get Waisted: 100 Addictively Delicious
Plant-Based Entrées* (by Tess Challis and Dr. Mary Clifton)

This easy dish is the epitome of Mexican comfort food. Creamy polenta is topped with all kinds of spicy, healthy goodies for a light, colorful, and satisfying entrée.

Polenta

> 3/4 cup dry polenta
>
> 3 cups water
>
> 3 tbsps nutritional yeast
>
> 3/4 tsp sea salt
>
> 3 medium-large cloves garlic, minced or pressed

Toppings

> Medium tomato, chopped
>
> 1/2 cup cooked black beans
>
> 1/4 cup **each**: diced green onions and chopped cilantro
>
> 1/2 medium avocado, chopped

Optional

> 2 tbsps minced jalapeno
>
> 1/2 fresh lime

1) Prepare all of the toppings and set them aside.

2) In a medium-large pot, place the polenta and water. Set to medium-high heat and bring to a boil, stirring with a wire whisk. Reduce heat to low and continue to whisk often until the polenta is thick. This should take about ten minutes.

3) Place the polenta in two bowls and top with the tomato, beans, onions, cilantro, and avocado. If desired, add the jalapeno and squeeze with lime juice. Serve.

GF/SF/Green (according to the guidelines in Tess's books)

Karina Inkster
Plant-based cookbook author and fitness coach
Karinainkster.com

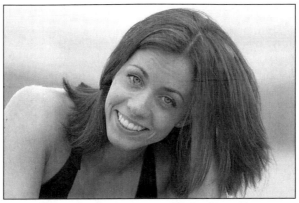

Karina Inkster
Photo by Elizabeth Lang

Karina is a self-proclaimed Professional Fitness Nut with a Master's Degree in Gerontology, specializing in health and aging. She offers in-person and online personal training, nutrition counseling, and lifestyle coaching. Her vegan cookbook and active living guide, *Vegan Vitality*, was published late 2014.

Green Machine Smoothie

We all know leafy greens are important to our health. To easily ramp up your leafy green intake, try drinking them!

> 2 cups plant-based milk
>
> 1/2 cup fresh or frozen spinach
>
> 1/2 apple, sliced
>
> 1 kiwi, peeled
>
> 1/2 cup cucumber, sliced
>
> 1/2 avocado

Place all ingredients into a blender and blend until smooth.

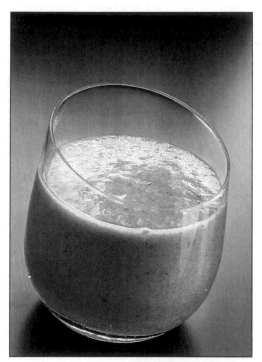

Photo by John Watson -
Imagemaker Photographic Studio

Orange, Carrot, and Ginger Smoothie

A refreshing combination of flavors that works well as a breakfast treat or afternoon snack.

> 2 cups plant-based milk (or 1 cup plant-based milk and 1 cup orange juice)
>
> 1 orange, peeled and segmented
>
> 1 medium carrot, chopped
>
> 1/2 inch piece fresh ginger
>
> 1/2 banana or 1/2 avocado

Place all ingredients into a blender and blend until smooth.

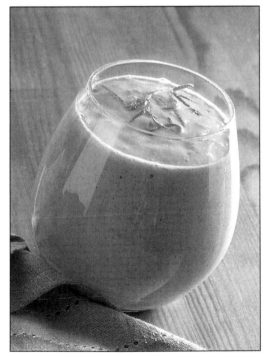

Photo by John Watson -
Imagemaker Photographic Studio

Rice Noodle Salad with Tofu, Water Chestnuts, and Herbs

This salad could easily be a meal in itself. It tastes like fresh spring rolls, but without the preparation work! If you can't find smoked or flavored tofu, marinate regular firm tofu in the dressing for 30 minutes before serving.

4 oz. dried rice noodles

Dressing

Juice of 2 limes

1/4 cup low sodium soy sauce

2 tbsp agave nectar

1 clove garlic, minced

1/2 tsp chili powder

1/4 tsp ground black pepper

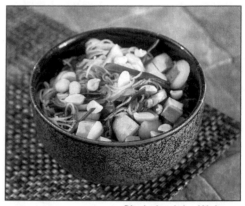

Photo by John Watson - Imagemaker Photographic Studio

Salad

1 pkg (8 oz.) smoked or flavored tofu, cut into small cubes

1 can (8 oz.) sliced water chestnuts, drained

1 1/2 cups purple cabbage, thinly sliced

1 cup cucumber, thinly sliced

1/2 cup white mushrooms, thinly sliced

3/4 cup fresh mint, chopped

3/4 cup fresh cilantro, chopped

1/2 cup fresh basil, chopped

1/2 cup roasted peanuts

Place noodles into medium saucepan and cover with boiling water. Let stand 3 to 5 minutes (until soft), then drain. Rinse with cold water.

In a small bowl, whisk together all dressing ingredients. In a large bowl, toss together all salad ingredients except peanuts. Add rice noodles and toss to separate and evenly distribute.

To serve, divide noodle and vegetable mixture among 4 bowls. Pour dressing over top and garnish with chopped peanuts.

Attila Hildmann
Bestselling cookbook author
attilahildmann.com

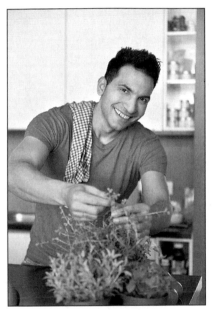

Attila Hildmann
Photo by Justyna Krzyzanowska

Attila Hildmann is Germany's No. 1 vegan cook. He believes that doctrines are out and that every vegan meal counts—and should taste great! He is a master of coming up with delicious and simple recipe ideas that even non-vegans are excited about. He has long been considered the "Jamie Oliver of Vegetarian and Vegan Cuisine" in the media. With his cookbooks, he has won numerous awards and sold over 700,000 copies.

Chili Crackers

Ingredients for 15 crackers

- 1 cup sunflower seeds (130 grams)
- 2 1/3 cups flax seeds (250 grams)
- 1 level tsp iodized sea salt
- 6 1/2 tbsps tomato paste (100 grams)
- 1 level tsp chili powder (to taste)
- 2 pinches turmeric

Preparation Time: Approximately 10 minutes plus approximately 45 minutes drying time in the oven or 6 1/2 hours of drying time in the dehydrator.

Grind sunflower seeds to a powder in a blender. Mix with the other ingredients in a large bowl and roll out on a dehydrator baking tray lined with a dehydrator non-stick sheet into a 11 1/4 x 8 1/4 inches (29 x 22 cm) rectangle. Alternatively, you can roll out the dough between two sheets of parchment paper on a baking sheet. To do this, put the dough on a sheet of parchment paper, flatten slightly using your hands, cover with a second piece of parchment paper, and roll the dough out with a rolling pin until you have a smooth, flat rectangle. If the rectangle isn't even on the edges, then mold it back together with your hands into the proper shape and roll over again with the rolling pin. Allow the crackers to dry in the dehydrator at 155°F (68°C) for approximately 6 1/2 hours or in the oven at 175°F (80°C) for approximately 45 minutes. Then cut the crackers into a diamond shape with a sharp knife.

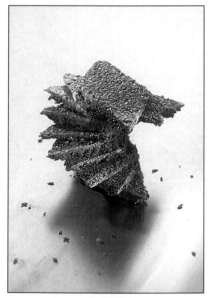

Photo by Johannes Schalk and Simon Vollmeyer

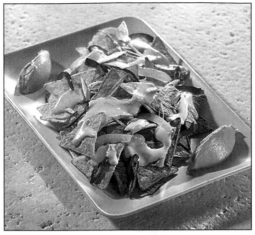

Shown here with tortilla chips
Photo by Johannes Schalk and Simon Vollmeyer

Avocados and Cashew Cheese Spread or Dip

Ingredients for 1–2 people

- 2 avocados
- 1 tbsp lemon juice
- Iodized sea salt
- Freshly ground black pepper
- 3 tbsps cashew butter (50 grams)
- 2 tbsps non-carbonated mineral water (1 ounce)
- 1 tsp nutritional yeast flakes
- 1/4 red bell pepper
- 1/4 yellow bell pepper
- 1 chili pepper
- 1 scallion

Preparation Time: Approximately 15 minutes halve the avocados, remove the pits, and spoon out about 1 1/2 cups (225 grams) of avocado. Purée with lemon juice until smooth. Season with salt and pepper.

Mix the cashew butter together with the mineral water and nutritional yeast flakes, and season with salt. Remove the core from the bell peppers, wash, and cut into fine strips. Wash and clean the chili pepper and scallion, and cut both into fine strips.

Whitney Lauritsen
Healthy Living Specialist and Creator of Eco-Vegan Gal
EcoVeganGal.com

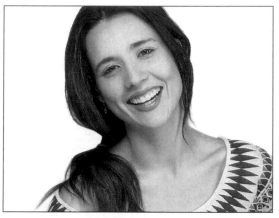

Whitney Lauritsen
Photo by Michel Hulsey

Whitney Lauritsen is the voice behind Eco-Vegan Gal, an online brand created to raise awareness about how to make healthy living choices and develop a planet-friendly lifestyle. Through videos, written articles and social media, Whitney shares simple lifestyle tips, product recommendations, easy recipes, inspirational interviews and more. This has resulted in a wildly successful YouTube channel, TV appearances, cover of Laika Magazine, and the Ed Begly Jr. Environmental Activist Award. She recently released the ebook, *Healthy, Organic, Vegan on a Budget,* and an accompanying meal plan service as guides on how to eat well with limited money and time.

Oil-free Kale Salad with Veggies & Seeds

This salad is incredibly easy to make and is a delicious example of how great veggies can be without oil or dressing. It's also a great way to feature kale in a dish. Though it is raw and unprocessed, keep in mind that the avocado and seeds add a significant amount of fat, so if you're trying to cut back on fat you may want to reduce the amount suggested in this recipe. From an eco-standpoint, this meal is wonderful because you can get everything without packaging!

> 1 bunch kale
>
> 1 medium or large avocado
>
> 1 medium or large carrot
>
> 1 medium tomato
>
> 1/2 medium white onion
>
> 1/2 lemon
>
> 1 tsp black pepper
>
> 1 tsp garlic powder
>
> 1 tsp hemp seeds
>
> **Optional**: Flax, sesame, and/or sunflower seeds

1) Break up leaves from kale and put into a bowl (compost the stems or use them to make broth)
2) Halve an avocado and scoop out 1/2 of it (or less to keep fat down, more to make it creamier) on top of the kale
3) Massage the avocado into the kale with your hands (make sure they're clean first!)
4) Dice the carrot and add into the salad bowl
5) Dice the tomato and add into the bowl
6) Halve the onion, dice and into the bowl
7) Massage everything until well combined
8) Squeeze lemon on top, and massage that in
9) Sprinkle on pepper, garlic and hemp seeds (as much as desired of each), and the other seeds if using
10) Optional: slice up the remaining half of the avocado and top on salad

Plate and enjoy!

Way Better Baked Mac 'n' "Cheese"

I'd like to say that a drop in temperature is responsible for the desire to eat comfort food, but let's be honest, when do you not want macaroni & cheese? OK, maybe it isn't that appealing on a super-hot day, but you can always serve it cold right? It's nearly impossible to resist the creamy texture and buttery taste. The only catch is that most mac 'n' cheese is loaded with oil, salt, soy and gluten, which can leave you feeling weighed down and bloated. Fortunately it doesn't have to be that way. This recipe puts a healthy spin on the classic favorite.

The "cheese" sauce is free of salt, oil, gluten and soy. The flavor is cheese-like and tangy (reminiscent of kale chips), the texture smooth and crunchy, and it is extremely filling. Inspired by a recipe in the *Forks Over Knives* cookbook, this dish is relatively low in fat and can be even more so if you cut back on the amount of cashews you use. Or, if you feel like indulging, double the amount of cashews to make it extra creamy!

> 1/2 cup raw cashews
> 1 cup nutritional yeast
> 1-2 garlic clove
> 1/2 large yellow onion
> 1 large red bell pepper
> 1 tbsp tahini
> 1 tbsp miso
> 1 tsp black pepper
> 1 tsp paprika
> 1 tsp crushed red pepper
> 1 tsp fresh lemon juice (or 1/2 a lemon)
> Gluten-free pasta of your choice

1) Soak cashews 1-6 hours, then remove from water (the longer you soak the better, but if you're short on time an hour is plenty)
2) Set oven to 350° F
3) Boil water on stove for pasta
4) Coarsely chop onion
5) Cut pepper open, wash seeds, then coarsely chop

6) Add cashews to blender along with chopped onions, pepper, and nutritional yeast. Blend well (add water if needed)

7) Add pasta to water and cook for 8-15 minutes depending on type

8) Dice garlic

9) Add garlic, tahini, miso, black pepper to taste, crushed red pepper to taste, and paprika to taste. Squeeze in half a lemon. Blend well. Adjust taste if needed by adding more of any of the above seasonings

10) Pour pasta into a casserole dish

11) Pour sauce on top and mix in well

12) Sprinkle on nutritional yeast and black pepper (paprika would be great too)

Put in oven and bake for 15-20 minutes

Mint Chocolate Coconut Tapioca Pudding

I've been trying to perfect chia seed pudding and have fallen flat so many times...until recently. I was inspired by my friend Vanessa Meier's recipe on her website, thegreengirlnextdoor.com, and with a few little adjustments to fit my diet and palate I came up with something insanely heavenly!

- 1 cup water
- 1 tbsp cashew* or almond butter
- 1 tbsp cacao powder
- 1 tbsp cacao nibs
- 1 tbsp unsweetened coconut flakes*
- 1 tsp coconut butter*
- 1/2 tsp vanilla
- 1/4 tsp stevia**
- 4-10 spearmint leaves
- 1/4 cup chia seeds

* Coconut & cashew may need to be omitted if you're on an anti-candida diet (depending on what stage you're on). You can also substitute the cacao for carob if need be.

** If you want to do it entirely raw, aren't on the anti-candida diet and/or don't like stevia you can use dates like Vanessa does in her recipe.

1) Blend everything except the chia seeds

2) Mix in the chia seeds

3) Put in the refrigerator for about 30 minutes (or more to make it thicker)

4) Take out and stir

5) Top with coconut flakes, cacao nibs, and a mint leaf

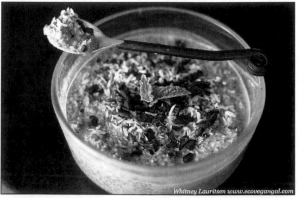

Whitney Lauritsen www.ecovegangal.com

Photo by Whitney Lauritsen

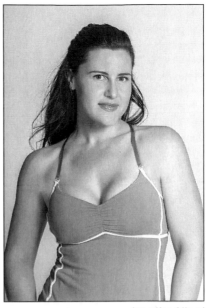

Jennifer Nicol
Photo by Lisa Luanne Photography

Jennifer Nicol
Health Coach, Plant-based
Registered Holistic Nutritionist,
and Certified Yoga Instructor
Lifestylepuravida.com

Jennifer's approach to nutrition is to keep it simple! Her meal plans are full of flavor, color, and texture. Jennifer encourages eating frequently, constantly introducing new foods and maintaining variety in the diet. She says, "A balanced body stems from a balanced mind and vice versa. It is essential we take fuel from clean, whole foods that provide natural energy to support the continuous movement and strength building of a healthy and strong body."

As a Registered Holistic Nutritionist, Jennifer feels it is necessary to not only eat a well-balanced diet but it is equally important to include regular exercise, stress management, self-inquiry and/or meditation practices as well as alternative medicine(s) into the lifestyle. During her studies at the Canadian School of Natural Nutrition, Jennifer rediscovered her passion for yoga and truly began to understand the plethora of holistic health benefits yoga has to offer. Jennifer successfully completed the 200-hour Yoga Teacher Training program to graduate simultaneously with the completion of her nutrition studies.

Outside of the yoga studio Jennifer enjoys short distance running 5-10km, cycling, strength training, and high intensity interval training. Jennifer is currently offering nutrition services, yoga class and wellness retreats in Canada, Costa Rica and Mexico. In addition to her business website listed above, learn more about her plant-based athlete lifestyle by visiting jennifernicol.com.

Crunchy Carrot & Celery Sauté served on Bean Wild Rice

Crunchy Carrot & Celery Sautee

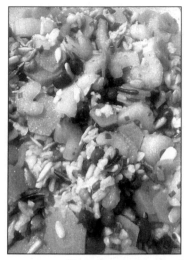

- 1 cup cooked and drained black beans or black organic soy beans
- 1/2 tsp fresh chopped or dried chives
- 2-3 carrots sliced into rounds
- 2-3 celery stalks cut sliced into 1/2 inch pieces
- 1-2 cloves of fresh garlic minced
- 1/4 small white onion minced
- 2-3 pinches sea salt or Himalayan salt
- 1/3 cup water
- Mung Bean wild rice

Photo by Jennifer Nicol

Set aside the beans. In a saucepan over medium heat, lightly sauté all ingredients (no beans) in 1/3 cup of water and a pinch of salt. In the last minute or two of preparation, gently fold the beans into the mixture in the pan, to warm up the beans. Remove from heat.

In a large bowl, mix celery carrot sauté and bean wild rice. Sprinkle with cayenne pepper and salt if desired. Serve hot.

Mung Bean Wild Rice

- 3/4 cup dry brown and wild rice blend (3 parts brown rice to 1 part black wild rice)
- 1/4 cup dry mung beans
- 1/4 tsp sea salt or Himalayan salt
- 1/4 cup raw sunflower or flax seeds (optional)
- 2 1/3 cups water

Bring water to a boil add salt, stir in all ingredients. Reduce heat to simmer. Keep the lid on throughout entire cooking time. Remove from heat after 50-55 minutes (could be a few minutes more or less, depends on stove top). Let stand for 10-12 minutes.

Serve hot.

Fresh Papaya Strawberry Mint Salad

1/4 large papaya cubed

8-10 strawberries sliced

1/2 cup of raspberries

1/2 cup blueberries

1 ripe banana

Juice of 1/2 fresh lemon

2 tbsps shaved unsweetened, unsulfured dried coconut

2 tbsps raw sunflower seeds or pumpkin/ sesame/ flax seeds

4-5 fresh mint leaves finely chopped into shreds

Gently fold ingredients together in a bowl. Chill for 20 minutes. Serve.

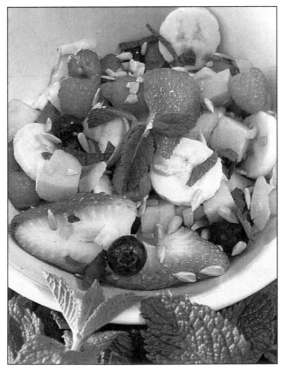

Photo by Jennifer Nicol

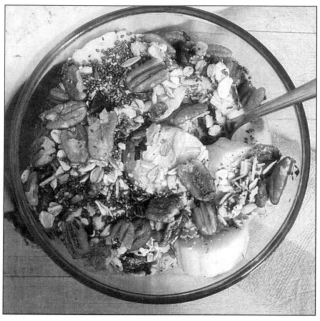

Photo by Jennifer Nicol

Pecan Banana Chia Bowl

3 tbsps chia seeds

2 tbsps dry oats

4-5 chopped Sayer cooking dates

1 tbsp raw pecans

1 tbsp sunflower seeds

1/2 tbsp flax seeds

1 small ripe banana sliced or substitute fresh berries or desired fresh fruit of choice

2/3 cup cold unsweetened almond milk

Mix all dry ingredients in a bowl, pour almond milk on top of mixture. Let stand for 3-5 minutes. Enjoy!

Quinoa, Baby Kale & Bean Salad in Citrus Garlic Herb Dressing

Individual Serving Size

> 1/2 cup of organic black soy beans drained and washed
>
> 1/3 cup of cooked and cooled quinoa
>
> 2 cups of organic baby kale washed
>
> 1/2 carrot cut into rounds

Toss all ingredients together in a bowl, add desired amount of citrus garlic herb dressing

Top with nuts and seeds if desired

Citrus Garlic Herb Dressing

> Juice of 1/2 fresh orange
>
> Juice of 1/4 fresh lemon
>
> 1-2 cloves of fresh raw garlic pressed or smashed and chopped finely
>
> 1-2 pinches of pink Himalayan salt
>
> 1 pinch cayenne pepper
>
> 1-2 sprigs of fresh chives or 1/4 tsp of dried chives

Whisk ingredients together and serve

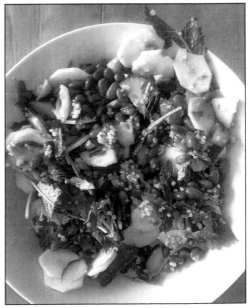

Photo by Jennifer Nicol

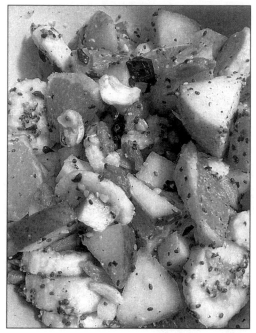

Photo by Jennifer Nicol

Goji Raw Chocolate Fruit Salad

1 organic Anjou pear cubed

1 organic Bartlett pear cubed

1 1/2 banana sliced

1 orange segmented and cubed

1/2 organic red delicious apple diced

2 tbsp dried Goji berries

2 tbsp chia seeds

1-2 tbsps raw cashews or nut of choice

1 tbsp finely chopped raw dark chocolate

Juice of 1/2 lemon

Mix all ingredients in a bowl. Chill for 20 minutes. Serve.

Sweet Buckwheat Groats & Banana Breakfast

1/2 cup buckwheat groats (not toasted)

1 1/4 cup water

1 1/2 tbsp organic raisins

2 pinches salt

1/4 tsp organic cinnamon

In a saucepan bring water to a boil. Add salt cinnamon, raisins and buckwheat groats. Reduce heat to minimum, place a lid on top and let simmer until almost all the water is gone. Keep the lid on and remove from heat. Let stand for 10 minutes before serving.

Top with sliced fresh banana or fresh fruit of choice and a sprinkling of cinnamon. Add nuts and seeds if desired.

Karen Oxley
Vegan Bodybuilding & Fitness Manager
VeganBodybuilding.com

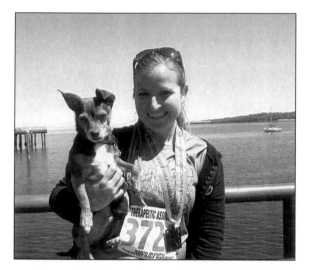

Karen is the content manager for Vegan Bodybuilding & Fitness on www.veganbodybuilding.com. She tours around North America on behalf of Vegan Bodybuilding & Fitness and prepares the majority of the meals that Robert Cheeke consumes to fuel his athletic success. She enjoys running and has completed half marathons in three different states (so far) including two in Oregon and two in Colorado. To see more of her recipes and prepared meals, follow her on Instagram at www.instagram/veganbodybuildingandfitness.

Basic Fruit and Green Smoothie

Smoothies are incredibly flexible. Use more or less of any ingredient, as you see fit.

1 large or 2 small oranges (peeled)

2 bananas

1 Granny Smith apple (minus the core)

2 cups of collard greens (or spinach)

1 cup water

2 cups of ice

Blend all ingredients together in high-powered blender.

Lemon Ginger Green Smoothie

1 lemon, peeled

2 inch piece of ginger root, peeled

2 bananas

2 cups of fresh spinach

1 cup water

2 cups of ice

Blend all ingredients together in high-powered blender.

3-Bean Tempeh Chili

This chili is so delicious, filling, and quick and easy to make. This is one of those dishes that tastes even better the next day, so you'll enjoy your leftovers. It makes a pretty big batch, so you'll have plenty to reheat for quick meals throughout the week. Or you can transfer this into smaller containers and store in the freezer until you are ready to defrost and reheat.

    2 cloves garlic
    1/2 onion, diced
    3 stalks of celery, diced
    3 carrots, diced
    1/2 green bell pepper, diced
    1 package tempeh, crumbled
    1 tbsp cumin
    1/2 tbsp chili powder (or to taste)
    1 1/2 cups (or 1 can) black beans, drained
    1 1/2 cups (or 1 can) pinto beans, drained
    1 1/2 cups (or 1 can) red kidney beans, drained
    1 can diced tomatoes (preferably fire roasted)
    1 can roasted green chilies
    1 cup of frozen corn
    1 cup of water

In a large pot, use enough water to sauté the garlic, onion, celery, and carrot. Sauté for about 5 minutes, until the vegetables have started to soften. Add the crumbled tempeh, cumin, and chili powder and continue to cook for a few more minutes, continuing to add water as needed to prevent burning. Add the remaining ingredients and simmer on low temperature until heated thoroughly.

Suggested toppings: avocado, fresh tomato, romaine lettuce, black olives, crushed red pepper flakes (if you like things more spicy).

Curried Chickpeas

1 yellow onion

2 cloves garlic

1 can lite coconut milk

4 cups (or 2 cans) garbanzo beans

1 can diced tomatoes (preferably fire roasted)

2 cups (or so) gold potatoes, cut into 1 inch pieces and boiled

1 tbsp tomato paste

1 tbsp curry powder

1 tbsp garam masala

½ tsp crushed red pepper flakes (or to taste)

2 cups fresh spinach

Sauté the onion and garlic in water, adding water as necessary to prevent burning. Add tomato paste and curry powder, mix well. Add remaining ingredients, except for spinach. Heat thoroughly, stirring occasionally. Add spinach and heat for 5-10 more minutes.

Serving suggestion: Serve over hot brown rice or with a whole wheat pita.

Kale Salad (Full Entrée)

4 cups of curly kale

Juice of one lemon

1 large avocado (or 2 small)

1 tomato, diced (or a handful of cherry tomatoes, halved)

1 1/2 cups (or 1 can) cannellini beans, drained

2 cloves garlic

1 package of tempeh, cut into bite-size pieces

1 tbsp cumin

½ tsp crushed red pepper flakes (or to taste)

Sauté the garlic in water, using enough to keep it from burning. Add tempeh, cumin, red pepper flakes, and more water to mix everything well. Cook until tempeh is browned and heated through. Add cannellini beans and heat through. Remove from heat and set aside.

Place the kale in a large bowl. Add the avocado and use your hands to massage the avocado into the kale. After several minutes, the kale will be softened. Add the lemon juice to the kale. Add the tempeh/bean mixture and the fresh tomato to the kale and mix well.

Mindy Collette
Vegan Fitness Model, Entrepreneur, Actress
MindyVegan.com

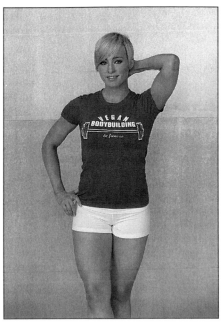

Photo by Melissa Schwartz
theveganrevolution.net

Mindy is a vegan athlete, singer/songwriter, dancer, animal rights activist, and fitness model. She currently resides in New York City where she provides private one-on-one personal training, practices yoga, and weight trains for fitness competitions. She auditions and goes to casting calls for magazines, films and theater work, pursuing her love for performing arts. Her ultimate goal is to be a voice for the voiceless, while sharing her passion for the compassionate, vegan lifestyle, because all lives are important and equal.

Sugar Cookie Smoothie

1 or 2 Medjool dates pitted

2 banana (frozen is ideal)

1/4 cup cashews

Cinnamon powder

1/2-1 cup nut milk (homemade preferred)

1/2 cup drained white cannellini beans

1/2-1 cup water (if you need more calories opt for 1 cup nut
milk to 1/2 cup water, or 1/2 cup nut milk and 1 cup water for
less fat and calories)

Ice

Optional: Add 1/4 cup raw oats for a more filling meal
shake. Also, pineapple or raspberries are a wonderful addition to this yummy drink!)

Red Velvet Cake Smoothie

1 small, or 1/2 large cooked, peeled red beet

1/2-1 cup nut milk

1 apple

1/2-1 cup water

1/4 tsp baking soda

1 tbsp cacao powder
Note: this can be substituted with cacao nibs.

1/4 cup macadamia, cashew, OR pecan nuts (raw, unsalted)

Ice

Blend!

Optional: 1-2 Medjool dates pitted

Kale Salad

Washed, torn/cut kale

1 carrot

1 bell pepper

1 lemon

1/2 avocado

Shelled edamame

1 tomato

Broccoli

Optional: Nutritional yeast

(Really any vegetable you love.)

Thoroughly rub both sides of the Kale leaves with lemon, toss all ingredients in a large bowl add seasoning as desired. I use black pepper, cayenne.

You don't need "dressing" because the lemon neutralizes the some-times bitter taste kale can have, and the nutritional yeast adds a nice "cheesy" factor. If you're open to it, add salsa. This is my all-time favorite salad!

Noodle Fest

1 package brown rice noodles (I prefer Tinkyada brand)

Zucchini

Tomatoes (fresh preferred, but if you are in a pinch and buy canned tomatoes or a sauce be sure to get a BPA-free can, or a jar without any added sugar or salt.)

Broccoli

Seasoning

Optional: Nutritional yeast

Walnuts or Pecans

Prepare noodles as package states.

Dice veggies, and set aside. If you have a Vitamix you can toss your whole tomatoes in with seasoning and make your own sauce rather easily. If not, you can just dice them up, put them in a sauté frying pan with water as needed and seasoning and simmer while noodles are cooking. Add veggies as desired.

Finely chop walnuts or pecans, add nutritional yeast, and season (I use black pepper, cayenne pepper, turmeric, and paprika). Top your spaghetti with Parma brand vegan cheese or add it to the sauce for a creamier outcome.

Robert Cheeke
Bestselling author, multi-sport athlete
VeganBodybuilding.com

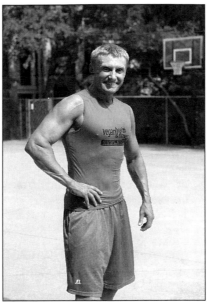

Photo by Brenda Carey

Robert is the founder and president of Vegan Bodybuilding & Fitness. He writes books, gives lectures all over the world, and maintains the popular website, VeganBodybuilding.com. He is a regular contributor to *Vegan Health & Fitness Magazine*, a multi-sport athlete, and has followed a plant-based diet for 20 years.

Super Basic Functional Recipes for Athletic Performance

Though I don't prepare a lot of my own food or follow many recipes, I do eat a lot of healthy whole foods to fuel my athletic endeavors and to support my health. The following are my pre-workout and post-workout recipes, though they could be consumed any time of day. This is as simple as it gets. For many, simple is best, or at least doable and practical. These are quick and easy. This is whole-food nutrition designed to work.

RC's Pre-workout recipes

Citrus Water

Create your own energy/electrolyte drink using whole foods.

Directions

Fill stainless steel water bottle with as much water as you like.

Cut as many lemons, limes, oranges, grapefruit or other citrus fruits as you like and squeeze the halves into your water bottle.

If the opening of your water bottle is too small, squeeze fruit into some other container first or use a funnel.

This is a great grip-strength and forearm muscle building exercise too. Compost the fruit peels or use any remaining parts of the fruits for future smoothies or salad dressings.

Drink and enjoy!

Seasonal Fruit Salad

Choose five of your favorite seasonal fruits and cut them into bite-size pieces and put them into a bowl for a natural pre-workout energy boost.

Directions

Select ripe, seasonal fruits and mix them into a large bowl for an anti-oxidant rich, high-energy producing, quick-digesting, pre-workout meal. Source fruits from a farmer's market or grow your own if possible. Try new fruits you've never had before. Mix it up and get creative.

Eat and enjoy!

Oatmeal with Berries

Create your own long-lasting, slow-releasing, complex carbohydrate breakfast to fuel you for the long haul. Complex carbohydrates like oats provide long, sustained energy and are a great fuel source before a workout.

Directions

Boil water, add desired quantity of steel cut oats, wait for oatmeal to be ready.

Add your favorite seasonal berries on top.

Add cinnamon or any other desired flavors for enhanced taste.

Add chopped bananas for additional calories for long-lasting fuel.

Eat and enjoy!

RC's Post-workout recipes

Yamwich

Use multiple large yams and your favorite legumes to make this awesome yamwich!

Directions

Slice up large yams into long flat strips resembling slices of bread.

Bake yams to desired texture. I prefer them to be fairly soft and pliable.

Prepare lentils, beans, or other legumes by boiling them on the stove.

Add desired legumes between two slices of baked yams. Bam! Yamwich!

Eat and enjoy!

Bean Me Up, Robby!

Select your three favorite beans and your three favorite greens

Directions

Soak, boil, or otherwise prepare your beans, ready to be eaten.

Steam your favorite greens.

Combine your favorite beans with your favorite greens and eat until you are full.

Enjoy!

Are You Stalking Me?

People tend to love the hairstyle on broccoli and cauliflower, among other stalky vegetables, but often forget about the stalk itself. Perhaps not as nutritionally dense as the "do," the stalk doesn't have to go to waste.

Choose your favorite cruciferous vegetables, and combine them with brown rice or quinoa for a post-workout meal worth stalking about.

Directions

Select your favorite cruciferous vegetables and steam them in sufficient quantities.

Prepare brown rice or quinoa in desired quantity.

Combine the vegetables with the grain or pseudo grain for a nutrition-packed meal that is great for lunch, dinner or after a workout.

Eat and enjoy!

Summary

Whether you try some of the intricate recipes with fancy photos, or combine beans and greens in a dish and give it a funny name, I hope the recipes in this chapter satisfy your hunger in your own sports nutrition ambitions. Cheers! Let's eat to grow! Or eat to lose, whichever fitness outcome you decide to choose.

Let's move on to the plant-based athletes, a community that is growing by the day. In the next chapter you'll get to know dozens of plant-based athletes leading the way toward a more compassionate future in sports.

– CHAPTER 11 –

Shredded Plant-Based Athletes

"I don't think of it as pushing myself. I think of it as letting myself go. It's easier for me to train than it is to not train, just because it's part of my lifestyle. I started it when I was fifteen and it's something that is really embedded in me."

— Brendan Brazier, former professional
ironman triathlete, elite runner

Back in the '90s I didn't know any other plant-based athletes, but today, most of my friends are plant-based athletes. We have over 200,000 members on our Vegan Bodybuilding & Fitness Facebook page, tens of thousands on other Facebook and Twitter pages, and of course, thousands of members on our primary website, www.veganbodybuilding.com. We sure have come a long way over the past couple of decades. The quote at the top of this chapter is from Brendan Brazier, one of the first plant-based athletes I ever heard of. When I became vegan in 1995 I hadn't even used the Internet and wasn't aware of anyone else living that lifestyle aside from a few high school friends who dabbled with veganism for short periods of time. When I got on the Internet years later I learned of a number of plant-based athletes I could count on one hand. As time went on I learned about Brendan and a handful of other athletes who seemed to be early adopters to what would later be a booming trend and shift in lifestyle for millions of people. Though Brendan was an early pioneer in the plant-based athlete lifestyle decades ago, he is still incredibly relevant today, pumping out one best-selling book after another and inspiring millions of people to change the world for the better through diet and exercise. I like to thank Brendan for his leadership and for being one of my all-time most inspirational role models. I've been very fortunate to work alongside Brendan for the past decade, and I owe a lot of my speaking tour and book writing success to the guidance he gave me. Though Brendan is one of the most popular names in the plant-based athlete world, as you're about to see, there are plenty of other high level athletes ditching animal products in favor of plants.

My company, Vegan Bodybuilding & Fitness, has sponsored a team of plant-based athletes over the years. We feature hundreds of plant-based athletes on our website, promote, and support hundreds of others, and have a plant-based athlete team we work very closely with to further the plant-based athlete message in mainstream culture. In addition to our Vegan Bodybuilding & Fitness athlete team, there are thousands of shredded plant-based athletes around the world. I highlight many of them in this chapter. You will read about athletes who have unique backgrounds, who have not only excelled in their chosen sports, but who embody the fat burning and building muscle themes I write about. All of them follow a vegan lifestyle, but not all of them eat exclusively whole foods. Many of the athletes you will read about are in fact getting shredded and building muscle on a primarily whole-food, plant-based diet. Others include processed foods and supplements. You can read more about each individual using their contact information provided with their bio. Many of these athletes have become some of my best friends over the years. The compassionate lifestylc we share has bonded us together as brothers and sisters working hard to make a positive difference in the world.

Which athletes follow a plant-based diet?

Historically, there have been plant-based athletes in a variety of mainstream sports that have reached the top of their industries. Athletes such as ten-time Olympic Medalist (including 9 Gold Medals), Carl Lewis, legendary tennis star, Martina Navratilova, four-time NBA champion, John Salley, and NHL great, Georges Laraque, to name a few, are synonymous with success in their sports and in popular sports culture. Their names are often synonymous with a plant-based diet too. The plant-based athlete community has embraced these sports greats for decades. They're not the only ones; they are just some of the most well known in our society. Ultra running champion, Scott Jurek is one of the best athletes on the planet, and Rip Esselstyn was one of the top ten professional triathletes in the world during his competition days, and was the number one swimmer in the sport. Brendan Brazier is a former professional ironman triathlete and elite distance runner, and Rich Roll has been considered one of the twenty-five fittest men in the world. Ruth Heidrich and Fiona Oakes are both champions and record-holders in some of the most grueling endurance races in the world. Mac Danzig is a professional mixed martial arts champion, and bodybuilder, Billy Simmonds, won the Mr. Universe title. Another bodybuilder, Jim Morris, won the Mr. America title, and is an outspoken vegan weightlifter at seventy-eight years old, still looking muscular and posing for photo shoots promoting the vegan athlete lifestyle. Patrik Baboumian is Germany's strongest man and has set world record lifts, including carrying the heaviest weight a human has every carried for a specific distance, and Laura Kline won the Short Course Duathlon World Championship in 2012. Even World Wrestling Entertainment (WWE) heavyweight champion, Daniel Bryan, is part of this elite plant-based athlete community. So is World Champion professional wrestler, Austin Aries. All of these athletes, and many other popular names, fuel their athletic success with plants.

As the overall population of individuals following a plant-based diet grows, so will the list of plant-based athletes. Today, we're seeing an array of elite athletes embracing a plant-based diet, including some of the most famous and successful athletes in the world, such as Serena and Venus Williams in professional tennis. NFL stars, NBA stars, professional soccer players, bodybuilders, weightlifters, and especially those involved in endurance running and mixed martial arts, have jumped on the plant-based bandwagon. This, of course, is good for the environment, good for the animals, and good for the plant-based community to have more names, faces, and successful role models to point to when discussing the plant-based lifestyle with the mainstream public. Even former heavyweight boxing champion, Mike Tyson, follows a plant-based diet. Like Mike, another boxing champion, who went undefeated for years at 30-0 (before a recent loss), Timothy Bradley, who defeated Manny Pacquiao, ending Manny's seven year undefeated streak, embraces a plant-based diet to fuel his unbelievable success, and has rarely ever experienced defeat in his sport.

Many athletes have arrived on the scene to help their recovery from injuries, help the prevention of injuries, and to capitalize on the basic benefits of having more energy, greater endurance, and faster recovery after exercise. Regardless of what brought many elite and professional athletes to the plant-based diet, they will provide more names to an already impressive group of successful plant-based athletes.

A list of notable, currently active athletes who have made it public that they follow a plant-based diet, include the following individuals (keep in mind this is just a sample list and we will keep an updated list on our website, www.veganbodybuilding.com, which you can reference anytime):

- Serena Williams, tennis champion
- Venus Williams, tennis champion
- Montell Owens, NFL running back
- David Carter, NFL defensive tackle
- Amare Stoudemire, NBA star
- Glen Davis, NBA star
- James Jones, two-time NBA champion
- Mac Danzig, MMA fighter
- Aaron Simpson, MMA fighter
- Mike Mahler, strength and conditioning coach
- Jon Hinds, strength coach and fitness equipment inventor
- Daniel Bryan, Champion pro wrestler
- Austin Aires, Champion pro wrestler
- Brendan Brazier, elite endurance runner
- Rich Roll, elite endurance runner
- Tim Van Orden, elite endurance runner
- Michael Arnstein, elite endurance runner
- Meagan Duhamel, Olympic figure skating silver medalist
- Alexey Voyevoda, three-time world champion arm wrestler and Olympic Gold medal-winning bobsledder
- Patrik Baboumian, Germany's strongest man
- Jeremy Moore, national level cyclist and speed skater
- Harley Johnstone, elite cyclist and runner
- Scott Jurek, ultramarathon champion
- Matt Frazier, runner
- Timothy Bradley, boxer
- Mike Zigomanis, hockey player
- Laura Kline, world champion duathlete
- Billy Simmonds, Mr. Universe

- Jake Shields, MMA fighter
- Nick Diaz, MMA fighter
- MaryJo Cooke Elliott, IFBB pro figure competitor
- Fiona Oakes, world champion ultra-runner
- Ruth Heidrich, endurance running champion
- Ellen Jaffe Jones, endurance running champion
- Torre Washington, champion professional bodybuilder
- Will Tucker, champion professional bodybuilder
- Jehina Malik, champion professional bodybuilder
- Frank Medrano, calisthenics specialist/fitness celebrity
- Daniel Negreanu, world's top poker player
- Phil Collen, martial artist and co-lead guitarist for Def Leppard
- Mike Malinin, ultra runner and former drummer for The Goo Goo Dolls
- John Joseph, triathlete and lead singer for the Cro-Mags
- Stic Man, athlete and singer for Dead Prez
- Leilani Munter, professional race car driver

The list of retired plant-based athletes, such as Carl Lewis and Martina Navratilova, is equally impressive. They helped pave the way for many of today's elite plant-based athletes and I honor them for the high standard they set. In addition to this list, there are thousands of other successful plant-based athletes in communities all over the world. Some may be relatively unknown but achieve high levels of success. For example, I watched a plant-based weight lifter friend of mine named Gabriel Hamel nearly set a world record in the deadlift for his weight class, yet because he doesn't have a strong online presence, his accomplishments are relatively unknown. This is true for thousands of plant-based athletes around the globe. Always remember that just because a certain individual isn't making headlines on ESPN or because they don't have a strong social media following, it doesn't mean they're not out there setting records and performing at high levels. I regularly meet people from around the world on my speaking tours who are outstanding plant-based athletes flying under the radar.

The following is a collection of plant-based athletes I interviewed specifically for this book. I deliberately listed their social media and website information so you can connect with them easily and directly. I sincerely appreciate each of them taking the time to share their plant-based lifestyles with me, and with you. Perhaps you will find some new role models in the ensuing pages. I know I have.

For ease of locating the specific page to find an athlete you're looking for to show friends to inspire others, I have listed these athletes alphabetically by last name. Bring on the shredded plant-based athletes!

Austin Barbisch

Birth year: 1968

Became plant-based: 2012

Height: 5'11"

Weight: 190 pounds (off season).
180 pounds (contest ready)

Sport: powerlifting, bodybuilding,
ultra-marathons, ultra rowing

Athletic highlights:

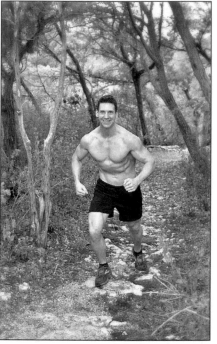

Photo by Christy Morgan

- 2nd Place – NASA power lifting meet

- 15 bodybuilding shows, placing 2nd nine times and winning twice

- 3:19.50 at the San Antonio Rock 'n' Roll marathon (Boston qualified)

- 1st Place – Run Like The Wind 12-hour foot race with 60.76 miles

- 1st Place – Run Like The Wind 24-hour race with 115.32 miles

- Two-time sub-24 hour Rocky Raccoon 100 mile foot race

- Completed a 33-mile ultra row in 4:40, and currently 1st place in Texas in the 500, 1000 and 2000 meter indoor rowing database division

- Inventor/developer of the PowerMarathon (powerlifting and marathon running on the same day with a combined performance scoring system)

- 1st Place – 2014 Naturally Super Show Masters Bodybuilding

Website: solidvegan.com

Facebook: facebook.com/austin.barbisch

Twitter: @AustinBarbisch

Austin's journey starts on the den floor of his mother's house. He was next to an empty bag of potato chips and a package of Oreos that had a few remaining after just pigging out. It was the summer of his sophomore year in high school and he was fat and daydreaming about how cool it would be to look like the solo flex guy, and race a bike in the Tour de France. He decided that he would embark on an 800-calorie a day diet consisting of two lean cuisine glazed chicken dinners, half a Hershey bar and a two-liter Diet Coke. A terrible diet, but his weight came off and his confidence went up. He started weight training when he turned seventeen by doing pull-ups in a door way and push-ups on the floor. He later joined a gym with a buddy to expand on new exercises.

At age twenty-four, he picked up running and five weeks later ran the Motorola marathon. He bicycled off and on during this time, and started competing in bodybuilding competitions (15 to date), and has taken on ultra marathon running and ultra rowing over the last several years. He is the #2 ranked indoor rower in the United States for his age group in the 500-meter distance and ranks in the top five in the 2000-meter and 5000-meter distances.

Switching to a vegan diet in 2012 drastically improved his performance and recovery from these intense events. He turned vegan for ethical reasons after knowing some vegan friends and seeing the movie *Earthlings*. Being vegan has really opened up his perspective on the way we treat our planet and the beautiful life forms who share it with us.

Ed Bauer

Birth year: 1979

Became plant-based: 1996

Height: 5'9"

Weight: 180 pounds

Sport: CrossFit

Athletic highlights:

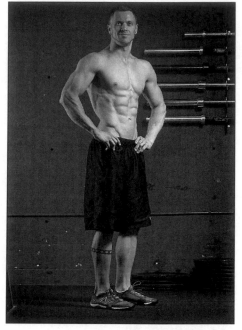

- May 2010 – 1st Place Novice Middleweight Bodybuilding Champion – NPC Bill Pearl High Desert Classic

- June 2011 – 4th Place Open Short Class – Washington State Natural Bodybuilding

Photo by Mark Rainha

- January 2012 – 34th Place out of 97 – Oregon CrossFit Winter Games

- March 2012 – 513th Place out of 1,584, Northwest Region – Reebok CrossFit Games Open (7,406 out of 25,083 Worldwide)

- August 2012 – 27th Place out of 73 – Oregon CrossFit Summer Games

- September 2012 – 23rd Place out of 39 – CrossFit X-Factor's Portland Throwdown

- July 2013 – 2nd Place out of 24, Men's Physique – INBF Naturally Fit Super Show

- July 2014 – 12th Place out of 25, Naturally Fit Super Show CrossFit Competition

Website: plantfitstrength.com

Facebook: facebook.com/pages/Plant-Fit-Strength/330510723629920

Twitter: @PlantFitXVX

Ed started weightlifting in 1995, with encouragement from his father, a competitive power lifter. This is when he learned the importance of exercise on overall health. He became vegan one year later, after learning about the inhumane practices that are involved in raising animals for food. Combining these two interests led to an understanding of plant-based nutrition and sports performance. In 2005, he began working at a small local gym. By taking care of himself through fitness and nutrition on a plant-based diet, awareness was spreading around him. It became clear that he could encourage compassion *and* well-being through his success on a plant-based diet. This has been his passion ever since.

In 2006, he became a Certified Personal Trainer. In 2010, he won his first bodybuilding competition. In 2011, he opened PlantFit Training Studio in Portland, OR. He operated that gym for two years before moving to the Bay Area of California in October 2013. He now runs the website www. plantfitstrength.com, trains multiple CrossFit classes at GrassRoots CrossFit in Berkeley, CA, as well as PlantFit BootCamps in both San Francisco and the East Bay. As a Fitness Nutrition Coach, he offers counseling on how to lose fat, increase muscle, and obtain optimal health and wellness on a plant-based diet. With over eighteen years as a vegan, eight years as a Certified Personal Trainer, and three years as a CrossFit Level 1 Coach, he can help you achieve your goals.

Arvid Beck

Birth year: 1982

Became plant-based: 2011

Height: 5'10"

Weight: Off-season, 187 pounds/
Competition, 172-176 pounds

Sport: Natural Bodybuilding

Athletic highlights:

- 3rd Place – German Vice-Champion and 3rd Place World Championships (Figure Class, NABBA/WFF)

Website: arvidbeck.de

Facebook: facebook.com/arvidbeckbodybuilder

Twitter: @ArvidBeck

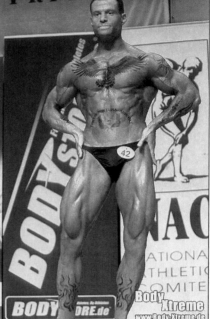

Photo by BodyXtreme.de

Arvid was born and raised in Düsseldorf, Germany, where he still lives today.

He first came in contact with bodybuilding when he did additional strength training for his martial art Ninjutsu. When he completed an internship for school in a gym in the year 2000, he immediately felt a strong passion for this sport, which led him to the decision to quit martial arts and focus fully on bodybuilding. Since then he has been training constantly and taken part in several competitions between 2006 and 2014.

After an earlier try to become vegan, he fully adopted a plant-based diet at the beginning of 2011. Although his decision was purely based on moral reasons, he came to the belief that it's also the healthiest way of eating and fits perfectly to a fitness and bodybuilding lifestyle.

His current diet is based on whole foods, with an emphasis on carbohydrates (up to 80 percent) and little fat (usually around 10 percent), and doesn't include any protein powders. His staples are grains, legumes, vegetables, and fruits.

For the future, he plans to compete in bodybuilding on a regular basis, and to spread the vegan message by being a positive example for other fitness enthusiasts.

Larry Bennett

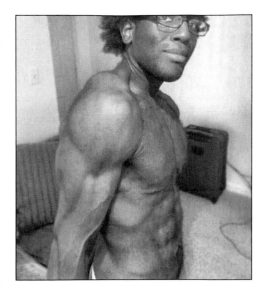

Birth year: 1986

Became plant-based: 2010

Height: 5'11"

Weight: 170 pounds

Sport: Street workouts
(calisthenics)

Website: larrybfit.com

Facebook: facebook.com/
larrybfit

Twitter: @larrybfit

Instagram: larrybfit

A whole-food, plant-based diet was essential to Larry's total body transformation. He had been obese for 90 percent of his life. At twenty-four, he was at his heaviest, tipping the scale at 320 pounds. After going vegan overnight, he was able to lose 135 pounds in just six months! Fast-forward three years later, he has now lost 150 total pounds! He does calisthenics training and operates his own health coaching practice where he works with clients who are focused on losing weight and toning their bodies. As Larry says, "Thanks for reading! Stay healthy!"

Tiffany Burich

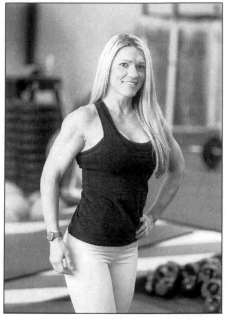

Birth year: 1981

Became plant-based: 2008

Height: 5'5"

Weight: 130 pounds

Sport: Bodybuilding (Figure & Fitness) and CrossFit

Athletic highlights:

- July 2013 – 3rd Place in Figure – INBF Naturally Fit Super-show (first bodybuilding show)

- September 2013 – 1st Place – CrossFit Challenge, Miami, FL

Photo by M-Magee Photography

- July 2014 – 3rd Place in Figure – INBF Naturally Fit Super Show

- July 2014 – 3rd Place in Fit Body – INBF Naturally Fit Super Show

Website: NoExcusesFitness.org & Plantbuilt.com

Facebook: facebook.com/tiffanyburich & facebook.com/veganpowerhousephysiques

Twitter: @TBurich

Tiffany is a vegan Figure Competitor, Fitness Model, Trainer, and Sponsored Athlete.

Born in Youngstown, OH, she moved to Miami, FL in 2002 to pursue fitness modeling and attend College. She is an ACE certified Personal Trainer, LV-1 CrossFit Trainer, has a B.S. in Exercise Science, and a B.S. in Biology (Pre-Med) from Florida Atlantic University. Her business is No Excuses Fitness & Nutrition (offering all types of fitness & nutrition plans) and she is part owner of Vegan Powerhouse Physiques (offering group online training). Since becoming vegan she has gained 20 pounds of muscle and has never felt better!

Chad Byers

Birth year: 1976

Became plant-based: 2011

Height: 6'4"

Weight: 212 pounds

Sport: Bodybuilding

Athletic highlights:

- 2012 – 1st Place – Naturally Fit Super Show, Men's Fit Model
- 2013 – 3rd Place – Naturally Fit Super Show, Men's Physique
- 2014 – 2nd Place – Natural Fit Super Show, Men's Physique

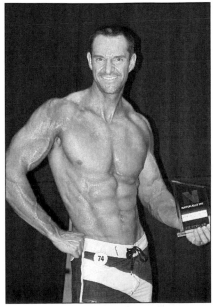

Photo by Tricia Kelly

Website: veganchad.com

Facebook: facebook.com/veganchad

Twitter: @veganchad

Instagram: theveganchad

Chad is a strength and conditioning coach and owner of Beyond Fit, a plant-based gym in Austin, TX. He trains all ages and fitness levels and promotes plant-based nutrition.

He has a degree in Exercise and Sports Science from Texas State University and has a minor in Health and Wellness. He is a certified Crossfit Kettlebell Instructor, TRX Trainer, and Hyperwear Sandbell Instructor. Chad is also certified in Plant-Based Nutrition through Cornell University and the T. Colin Campbell Foundation.

Chad is a member of the Vegan Bodybuilding & Fitness Team, a member of the PlantBuilt Team, a Clean Machine sponsored athlete, as well as a featured athlete and contributor for Vegan Bodybuilding and Fitness. He has written articles on health and fitness topics for *Naturally Fit*, *InFluential*, and *Vegan Health and Fitness* Magazines.

Richard Campbell

Birth year: 1976

Became plant-based: 2013

Height: 6'0"

Weight: 205 pounds

Sport: Bodybuilding

Athletic highlights:

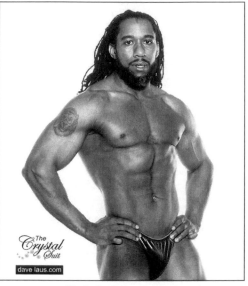

Photo by Dave Laus - DaveLaus.com

- 2011 – IDFA World Championships & Pro (International Drug Free Athletes)

- November 2011 – 3rd Place – Bodybuilding Heavyweight Novice category

- 2012 – WBFF World Championships (World Beauty Fitness & Fashion)

- August 2012 – 6th Place – Muscle Model Open category

- 2013 – IDFA World Championships & Pro (International Drug Free Athletes)

- November 2013 – 7th Place – Bodybuilding Heavyweight Open category

Website: livityfitness.com

Facebook: facebook.com/#!/RichardCampbellVeganBodybuilder

Twitter: @livityfitness

Richard was born on April 7, 1976 in Toronto, Ontario, Canada to parents of Jamaican heritage. He started competing in bodybuilding competitions in November 2011, where he placed 3rd in the men's heavyweight category at a natural bodybuilding contest. He became a vegan on April 7, 2013, his thirty-seventh birthday. He decided to become a vegan for moral, ethical, and spiritual reasons. "Eating vegan feels right for the mind, body, and soul," he said. There are many reasons why he became a vegan, but the main reason was for his spiritual beliefs. He is a Rastafarian and in the

Rastafarian faith, they believe that your body is a temple and death should not enter your temple.

Being a vegan is a "Livity" way of life, according to Richard. "Livity means life, Livity means love, Livity means loving other people in the same way you love yourself. Livity means being connected to the life source, the earth and everything that sustains it," he added. He is very driven when it comes to fitness and living a healthy lifestyle. It's a way of life for Richard and he embraces it. Fitness and living a healthy lifestyle is a Livity for him. His favorite *vegan* quote: "Vegan food is soul food in its truest form. Soul food means to feed the soul. And, to me, your soul is your intent. If your intent is pure, you are pure." — Erykah Badu

Mindy Collette

Birth year: 1986

Became plant-based: 2010

Height: 5'6"

Weight: 127 pounds

Sport: Strength training, figure/ bikini competitor, dancer

Athletic highlights:

- 2009 – 2nd Place – NPC Figure Division

- 2013 – 4th Place – Naturally Fit Super Show Bikini/Fit Model Division

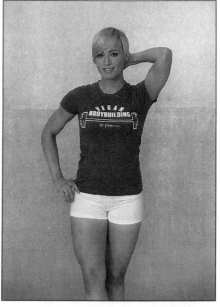

Photo by Melissa Schwartz - theveganrevolution.net

- 2014 – 2nd Place – Naturally Fit Super Show Fit Model Division

Website: mindyvegan.com

Facebook: facebook.com/mindyvegan

Twitter: @MindyVegan

Instagram: MindyVegan

Mindy is a vegan athlete, singer/song-writer, dancer, and animal rights activist, but she hasn't always been all of these things. From Mindy's humble beginnings in a very small rural town, in the southern Oregon forests she called home, sparked her adventurous creativity from a young age. With no neighbors for at least a mile, and being the youngest of four much older siblings, her best friends were her black lab, Patty, and her imagination. Growing up, her mother would drive her 50 minutes—each way—to dance classes or musical theatre rehearsals 5-6 days a week from around five years of age until 2003, at 16 when she graduated high school and moved away to college. Throughout her college years Mindy continued to pursue dance, until her early twenties when she discovered the challenge of weightlifting.

In late 2008 she saw a poster for a figure competitor guest poser for an upcoming NPC bodybuilding competition, and knew at once what she needed to do. On May 2, 2009 Mindy competed in her first NPC figure competition and took second place in her division. What made that day all the more exciting, however, was that she met Robert Cheeke backstage, and, in turn, first learned of veganism. Mindy competes as a member of team Plant Built, and is a vegan for more than four years. She currently resides in New York City where she provides private one-on-one personal training, practices yoga, and weight trains for fitness competitions. She auditions and goes to casting calls for magazines, films and theater work, pursuing her love for performing arts. Her ultimate goal is to be a voice for the voiceless, while sharing her passion for the compassionate, vegan lifestyle, because all lives are important and equal.

Simone Collins

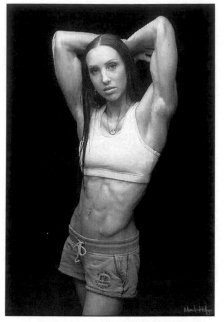

Birth year: 1986

Became plant-based: 2009

Height: 5'6"

Weight: 121 pounds

Sport: Figure, Bodybuilding

Athletic highlights:

- 2013 IFBB – 4th Place – Australian Amateur Grand Prix Figure Novice

- 2013 IFBB – 3rd Place – Victorian State Titles Figure Novice

*Photo by Mark Hillyer Photography -
markhillyer.com.au*

- 2014 IFBB – 6th Place – Australian Amateur Grand Prix Figure Novice

- 2014 IFBB – 2nd Place – O'Mara Classic and World Qualifier

Website: simicollins.com

Facebook: facebook.com/simi.monique

Instagram: simi_collins

Simone is a vegan figure athlete and competitor who works as a graphic designer, and is also studying for her personal training certifications.

She has been vegan since 2009 and meat-free since 1999. She began weight training in 2010 and recently started competing in bodybuilding competitions in the 'novice figure' division.

Her choice to go vegan was completely ethical. She stopped eating meat due to her love for animals and a desire to live more compassionately, however thanks to campaigns run by Animal Liberation Victoria (www.alg.org) she became aware of the cruel, immoral, and unethical treatment and killing of animals that exists throughout all animal industries, even the dairy and egg farming, and those claiming to be organic, biodynamic, or free-range.

Simone trains 5-6 days a week, mainly with weights. Training for and competing in bodybuilding shows is not only her passion, but she also uses competing as her own form of activism—an opportunity to break the "skinny weak vegan" stereotype, and to prove to people what is really achievable on a natural vegan diet. The belief in consuming meat, dairy, and animal-derived supplements is so entrenched in sports, particularly bodybuilding, and she hopes to be able to show that this is not the case—that achieving your health and fitness goals is not only possible on a compassionate, plant-based diet, it is ideal.

Lauren Goebel

Birth year: 1991

Became plant-based: 2011

Height: 5'1"

Weight: 105 pounds

Sport: Triathlons, half marathons

Athletic highlights:

Half Marathons:

- 2013 – Strongsville Fall Classic
- 2012 – Miami Beach Half Marathon

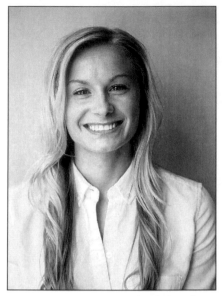

Photo by Amber Gress

Triathlons:
- 2009 – Florida Gulf Cost University Triathlon
- 2011 – Cleveland Triathlon

Website: livelikelu.wordpress.com/

Facebook: facebook.com/lauren.goebel.5

Twitter: @laurengoebel2

Lauren is in her early twenties and has been vegan for over three years. She is currently a senior at Florida Gulf Coast University, majoring in exercise science. She has been accepted to Naturopathic Medical School where she will start on her holistic journey to become a Naturopathic Doctor. Lauren has completed two triathlons, finishing in second and fourth in her age group. She has also completed two half-marathons, finishing in second and eighth in her ago group. Lauren competed in her first USPA powerlifting meet on March 29, 2014 competing in the 105-pound weight class for both the raw open and raw juniors divisions. She placed first in the raw open division. She qualified in the junior division for World Championships at the Master Level and will be competing at World Championships in November 2014. She also set the American record in the junior division for her deadlift, lifting 288 pounds. She broke all of the state records in Ohio for both the open and junior division.

Lauren will continue to train as a powerlifter focusing on speed work, which will ultimately help her to gain faster times in her next triathlon.

Edward Goins

Birth year: 1980

Became plant-based: 1996

Height: 5'10"

Weight: 194 pounds

Sport: Rugby

Website: totalexhaustionfitness.com

Facebook: facebook.com/
totalexhaustion

Twitter: @veganprince

Edward has been a vegan for the past seventeen years. A vegetarian since age seven, he has always had a passion for animal rights and fitness. His goal is to be an example of how one can live a balanced, healthy, and invigorating lifestyle that does not impose on the sanctity of animal's lives. Fitness was a logical progression from his naturally active routine—competing in cycling, recreational surfing, competitive rugby and semi-professional football—Edward has always pushed his body to new limits. He takes pride in his heavily sculpted physique and relishes any opportunity to share with someone that he is, in fact, vegan. He utilizes the same discipline from his vegan diet to fuel his high intensity workouts and encourages anyone who is involved in fitness to think as critically about their diet as they do about their training.

Melissa Hauser

Birth year: 1980

Became plant-based: 2012

Height: 5' 2"

Weight: 125 pounds (off-season); 115 pounds (competition)

Sport: Women's Figure, Bodybuilding (NPC)

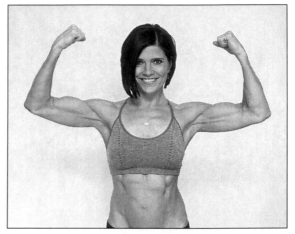

Photo by Sarah Lechner
sarahreneephoto.zenfolio.com

Athletic highlights:

- August 2013 – 2nd Place Novice, Short; 5th Place Open; Class B – The Warrior Classic
- October 2013 – 1st Place Novice, Short; 1st Place Novice, Overall; 1st Place Open, Class B – The GNC Natural
- July 2014 – 2nd Place - Colorado State Figure Championships
- July 2014 – 2nd Place Naturally Fit Super Show Figure Division

Website: blogger.com/profile/01241410816809750169

Facebook: facebook.com/plantpoweredhauser/

Instagram: @PlantPoweredHauser

Melissa was always fairly athletic, taking part in various sports in high school and teaching aerobics in college. But it wasn't until after she had her son in 2012 that Melissa really became focused on fitness and health. Like many women post-partum, she fit in workouts where and when she could, and dropped most of her baby weight working out to DVDs in her living room. A few months later, she joined a local Denver, CO gym, where she fell in love with weightlifting and gained an interest in competing in the bodybuilding industry.

A vegetarian since 2009 and vegan since 2012, Melissa faced skepticism and doubt from her trainer that she could be competitive in a sport dominated by animal-protein fueled diets. Yet she pursued the stage and placed in each NPC show she entered in 2013 and had two runner-up finishes in 2014.

Melissa is passionate that clean, plant-based eating is the solution to myriad global problems. She practices compassion and kindness in her life, and hopes that her success in the world of competitive bodybuilding will continue to dispel myths about plant-based eating. Melissa lives in Denver with her son Nolan, and husband David.

Attila Hildmann

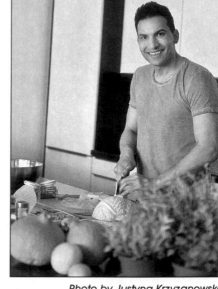

Birth year: 1981

Became plant-based: 2000

Height: 5' 10"

Weight: 150 pounds

Sport: Ironman Triathlon, Fitness

Athletic highlights:

- 70.3 Ironman Wiesbaden
- 70.3 Ironman Berlin

Website: bjv-books.com

Facebook: facebook.com/
attilahildmannpage

Photo by Justyna Krzyzanowska

Twitter: @attila_hildmann

Attila lost more than 77 pounds since he became vegan. Before that, he had tried almost every diet on the planet. None of them had any lasting success. Back then, as an overweight couch potato, he resolved that one day he would be on the cover of *Men's Health* magazine. His goals seemed crazy to those around him at that point. But when you look at him today and compare with the photos from thirteen years ago, which can be seen on his Facebook page, you see a transformation that is simply amazing.

Today, he has multiple Ironman Triathlons behind him and has the fitness level and appearance that he had dreamed about back then. He achieved this because he kept the finish line in sight, true to his motto, "If you reach for the stars, you'll often at least land on the moon." And *Men's Health* is now within reach.

In his bestselling book, *Vegan for Fit*, Attila shows what people can achieve in 30 days with a total reset of their body and spirit. The amazing improvements in fitness, health, and appearance that over 100,000 challengers have made speak for themselves. The Challenge is not a diet, but rather an extremely healthy way of eating that is simple to carry out, satisfying, and delicious. And on top of all that, it is easy to lose weight and build muscles this way.

JoJo Hulett

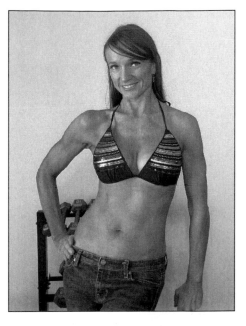

Birth year: 1971

Became plant-based: 2007

Height: 5' 6.5"

Weight: 128-130 pounds

Sport: Weightlifting, TRX, lead/ instruct circuit training classes, and occasionally run 5K races

Facebook: facebook.com/ VeganFitJojo

Twitter: @JojoHulett

JoJo began eliminating animals from her diet shortly after high school. She could not see a real distinction between her pets, and what was on her plate. By 1991, she was vegetarian. She started weight training with a friend in 2000, but their lives took different paths and she lost her motivation to train alone. Fast-forward seven years...a big fan of cheese, she was horrified by what she learned about the dairy industry and immediately became vegan. As she began to battle an extra 10 pounds in her 30s, her interest in weight training was renewed. It was then that she found the book, *Vegan Bodybuilding & Fitness*. This was a pivotal point in her life. She cried as her mind soaked up Chapter 8, "Turning your Bodybuilding Success into a Form of Effective Activism and Outreach." She decided at that moment that she was going to work to make people take notice, and change their negative perception about vegans being weak and sickly. The author's words had switched on a light in her head—a very bright light that continues to power her drive to be an inspirational, strong and healthy walking billboard for farmed animals.

Tricia Kelly

Birth year: 1985

Became plant-based: 2012

Height: 5' 8"

Weight: 150 pounds

Sport: Weightlifting

Website: beyondfitaustin.com/
tricia-kelly.html

Facebook: facebook.com/vegantk

Twitter: @tkofitatx

Instagram: tkofitatx

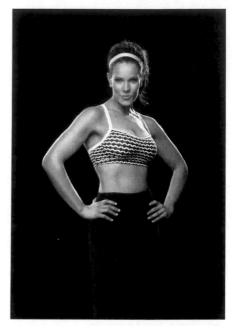

*Photo by Melissa Schwartz -
theveganrevolution.net*

Tricia is a plant-based athlete and fitness coach at Beyond FIT in Austin, TX. She has been vegan since 2012 and has transformed her life, mindset, and body by losing over 125 pounds over the past few years.

As a woman who has struggled with her weight and body image, Tricia understands many of the things that hold people back from turning their intentions into actions. She believes that one must maintain a positive mindset and vision while taking action toward specific goals. Tricia advocates a plant-based diet and believes that healthy food should be used for fueling the body.

Tobias Klingl

Birth year: 1988

Became plant-based: 2012

Height: 5' 7"

Weight: 160 pounds

Sports: Bodybuilding, Wrestling

Facebook: facebook.com/tobias.
klingl.56

Twitter: @TobiasVKlingl

Instagram: veganvitness

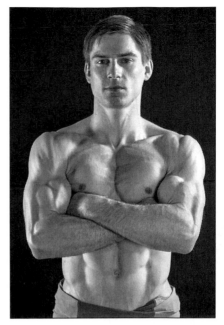

*Photo by Falko Werner -
picture4u.de*

Tobias started wrestling when he was seven years old. Even at this age he loved to do push-ups, pull-ups, and sit-ups. As he got older, and further along in his wrestling development, it was beneficial to have more strength than his opponents. For that reason, he started functional weight training in the gym at the age of fifteen. The more he trained in the gym the more he loved weight training, and at the age of twenty-two he changed his focus from wrestling to bodybuilding. He also became more interested in nutrition and what his body really needs to build up muscles and to stay healthy. He started bodybuilding as a meat eater and it took a few months for him to become aware of what we, as a society, are doing to the animals. As a result, he became a vegetarian in 2011 and vegan in 2012. Being vegan and building up muscles was never a contradiction to Tobias. Since he became vegan he increased his strength, built up muscles, and reduced body fat. He said that becoming vegan was one of the best decisions of his life.

Elena Kulakovska

Birth year: 1982

Became plant-based: 2012

Height: 5' 6"

Weight: 120 pounds

Sport: Yoga and cycling

Athletic highlights:

- Yoga certified

Website: kulhealthyyou.com

Facebook: facebook.com/
   KulHealthyYou

Twitter: @KulHealthyYou

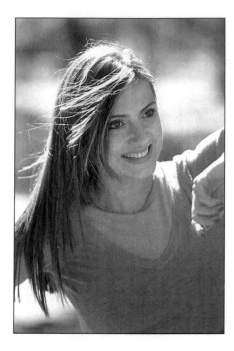

Elena is a certified holistic health coach helping athletes improve their fitness through nutrition. Through individually tailored programs, she also helps people make healthier lifestyle choices that stick for the long term. Her VIP day retreats make it possible for her busy clients to transform their lives in just one day of coaching. When working with Elena, together you will explore recommendations based on your intentions and lifestyle goals, ultimately leading you to live a healthy and fulfilling life while saving money in the long term.

Check out her website for awesome tips on nutrition as well as her VIP day coaching programs.

Aaron MacNeil

Birth year: 1976

Became plant-based: 2009

Height: 5' 7"

Weight: 185 pounds

Sport: Hockey, basketball, soccer, football and bodybuilding

Photo by Victoria Prince

Athletic highlights:

- Specializes in interval training and high intensity weight training with strong interests in hiking and climbing

Facebook: facebook.com/groups/macneilcustomfirness/

Twitter: @aaronmacneil1

Aaron is a dedicated family man who is devoted to raising healthy children and sharing his journey of everyday health and fitness to help others. He is also passionate and creative in the kitchen. His lucky family is always treated to new and delicious concoctions!

Aaron's journey started five years ago when he came to the realization that if he wanted to live a long fulfilling life he needed to change his lifestyle habits. After going vegan he lost a considerable amount of weight and his health issues simply faded away. He now spends a lot of time researching food to learn how food affects the body. To keep things interesting, he is always studying different exercise styles, then testing and altering them, to produce the fastest and most effective results that render the quickest body transformations. His favorite training includes a combination of high intensity weightlifting and interval training.

Aaron believes a combination of clean eating, exercise, and a calm mind can lead to true wellness and happiness. Although steadfast in his desire for optimal health and fitness, he is content knowing there is no destination, but that he is on a life-long journey.

Giacomo Marchese

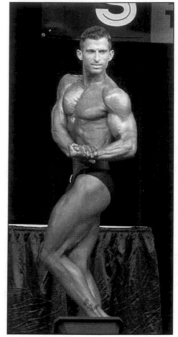

Birth year: 1980

Became plant-based: 2004

Height: 5' 10"

Weight: 180-200 pounds

Sport: Bodybuilding

Athletic highlights:

- 2002 – 1st Place – INBF (Brooklyn, NY) All Natural Bodybuilding Fitness Explosion
- 2009 – 6th Place – INBF (Phoenix, AZ) Best of the West Championships
- 2009 – 2nd Place – INBA (Clackamas, OR) INBA Northwestern USA

Photo by Donovan Jenkins

- 2013 – 3rd Place – INBF (Austin, TX) Naturally Fit Super Show
- 2014 – 4th Place – INBF (Austin, TX) Naturally Fit Super Show

Website: VeganProteins.com and PlantBuilt.com

Facebook: facebook.com/VeganProteins

Twitter: @VeganProteins

Instagram: Leanandgreen719

After watching a friend almost lose their life to a heart attack at a young age, Giacomo decided he wanted to help. He started to look into what causes disease and through research, he found that a plant-based diet was the best way to prevent and reverse heart disease. Going vegan also proved to be the best way to fuel his body as an athlete, and Giacomo has been able to achieve exceptional results in his sport of bodybuilding.

Being vegan took on meaning for Giacomo and it became about living a compassionate and cruelty free lifestyle. He has since devoted his life to leading by example, with hopes of inspiring others to embrace vegan-ism. In late 2012, Giacomo and his fiancé Dani Taylor reached out to their colleagues, who agreed to work together and form a vegan muscle team. Dani and Giacomo co-founded PlantBuilt.com and became the team captains, turning their idea into a reality! Giacomo is active in his sport and plans on competing for the long term, so he can show others what is truly possible by going vegan.

Ryan Nelson

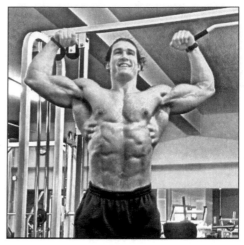

Birth year: 1988

Became plant-based: 2012

Height: 6' 4"

Weight: 250 pounds

Sport: Previously football/
currently bodybuilding

Athletic highlights:

- 2010 – Honorable Mention NSIC Defensive End
- 2011 – IFL Team Captain
- 2013 – Completed a 605-pound deadlift
- 2014 – 2nd & 3rd Place – Super Heavyweight Bodybuilding Competition

Website: alphafitnessmn.com

Facebook: facebook.com/NPCBodybuilderRyanNelson

Twitter: @AlphaD307

Growing up, Ryan wanted to be a football player. He worked hard and received a football scholarship from the University of Mary in Bismark, ND. He graduated with a BS in Sport Management and went on to play professional football. Later he would pursue weightlifting and eventually bodybuilding. He deadlifted over 600 pounds while training with his lifting partner, Matt Kolden, and has been a fan of the hardcore gym chain, MetroFlex, where he had some of his most memorable lifts. Today he is a personal trainer and competitive bodybuilder.

When Ryan became vegan nearly two years ago, he described it as "seeing the light," and said that a vegan lifestyle has truly changed his life in positive ways. His philosophy is that hard work and patience will always persevere. To Ryan this means focusing on muscular strength, physical endurance, nutrition, flexibility, rest, and mental stimulation. "I really emphasize the little things because in the end just having a couple percent more optimal health over a period of time will make the difference in being number one or number two," he explained.

Monica Parodi

Birth year: 1973

Became plant-based: 2010

Height: 5' 7"

Weight: 122 pounds

Sport: Bodybuilding

Athletic highlights:

- P90X2 Cast Member
- P90X Military Tours Cast Member
- P90X/QVC TV Show Cast Member

Website: monicaparodi.com

Facebook: facebook.com/thenutritionista

Twitter: @monica_parodi

Instagram: monica_parodi_

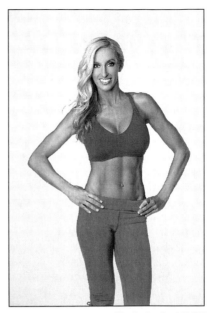

Photo by Todd Vitti

Monica is an internationally published author, fitness enthusiast, Ph.D. student, and nutrition expert. Her proudest accomplishment to date is being the mother of three small children—including twins. Monica's holistic approach to health, wellness, and beauty has been a source of inspiration for countless people seeking healthier, happier lives. Monica makes fitness and being a plant-based athlete an integral part of her life. It's important that she lives a life that will leave a legacy of health and fitness to her family and those that cross her path. Her true passion is teaching families to thrive on whole-foods nutrition. Monica isn't your typical athlete as a 40+ year-old mother of three, and that in itself speaks to the power of training on a plant-based diet. You can learn more about Monica's fit vegan lifestyle in her column in *Vegan Health & Fitness Magazine*.

Elana Priesman

Birth year: 1977

Became plant-based: 2012

Height: 5' 1.5"

Weight: 137-139 pounds

Sport: HIIT cardio and
  Weightlifting

Athletic highlights:

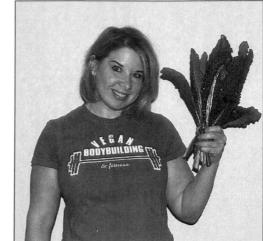

- July 2014 – 4th Place –
  Naturally Fit Super Show Transformation

Website: plantsformation.com

Facebook: facebook.com/plantsformation

Twitter: @plantsformation

Elana is a woman who struggled with weight and food issues her entire life. She spent over twenty-five years trying to connect the pieces of a puzzle that could make her manage her weight sanely. She is a mother to an active toddler, is an excellent role model giving her daughter an early start to a healthy vegan lifestyle, and is proud her child can name every single fruit and vegetable out loud in the supermarket.

She became vegan after a health scare that made her question whether she would be around to watch her baby grow up. She decided to become accountable to her actions and change her food choices. Since adopting a plant-based diet, Elana has dropped over 80 pounds, but gained a wealth of knowledge that she is passionate about sharing to help inspire others to change their lives through her Facebook page, Plantsformation.

Elana is co-owner in a company that manufactures natural and safe skin and hair care products for babies and children, Bathtime Baby & Bathtime Kids. She is knowledgeable about toxins in personal care products, and their affect on the body, and realized that food and nutritional choices were equally important.

Marzia Prince

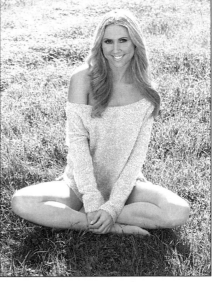

Birth year: 1974

Became plant-based: 2009

Height: 5' 9"

Weight: 135 pounds

Sport: Bodybuilding, yoga, barre, aerial silks, and TRX

Athletic highlights:

- 2007 – Winner – Ms. Bikini Universe Winner
- 2008 – Winner – FAME Bikini Championship Winner

Photo by Wade Livingston - wadelivingston.com

- 2009 – Winner – Jr. National Bikini Champion and IFBB Pro

Website: MarziaPrince.com and HealthyHousewives.com

Facebook: facebook.com/marzia.fitness

Twitter: @MarziaPrince

Marzia became an international fitness supermodel in her 30s. She is a fitness expert, life coach, competitor, and a published holistic health writer. She is one of the pioneers who brought the bikini fitness body type to the bodybuilding world. She has graced several fitness and bodybuilding covers that include *Fitness Magazine, Natural Muscle Magazine, Iron Man Magazine, Muscular Development Magazine, Planet Muscle Magazine,* and many more. At thirty-two years old, she signed with Gaspari Nutrition, which catapulted her fitness career. She went from fitness trainer to fitness supermodel overnight. After seven years, Marzia hung up her competition heels in 2010 to focus on her health blog, The Healthy Housewives. At thirty-eight years old, Marzia signed on with SunWarrior as a spokesmodel for the holistic health community. Marzia is an ambassador on holistic health and wellness. She believes in living a cruelty-free life from what she eats to what she wears for fashion.

Joel Rosario

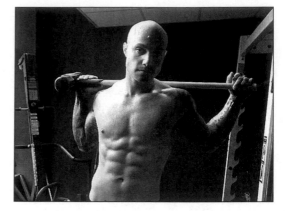

Birth year: 1986

Became plant-based: 2011

Height: 5' 6"

Weight: 168 pounds

Sport: Olympic Lifting, CrossFit, Long Distance Running

Athletic highlights:

- 2012 – Stone Mill Ultra Marathon, CrossFit Athlete

Facebook: facebook.com/NotYourAverageVegan

Joel is a twenty-eight-year-old firefighter/paramedic with first hand exposure to knowing how easily life can be taken for granted in regards to health. Joel is passionate about sharing his love for plant-based food and is devoted to destroying the misconceptions of how the general public perceives plant-based athletes. Aside from saving lives through his career as a firefighter, Joel continuously reminds us of how easy it is to adapt to your surroundings both socially and physically while committing to a plant-based diet. Being of Latin decent, he has adapted both his culture and tradition into his plant-based lifestyle. Aside from his strict training regimen, Joel also trains other athletes and is currently a USA-W Olympic Lifting Coach and a CrossFit Level 1 Coach.

Roger Smith

Birth year: 1978

Became plant-based: 2002

Height: 6' 2"

Weight: 220 pounds

Sport: Bodybuilding, Crossfit, and Basketball

Athletic highlights:

- 2014 – 4th Place – Naturally Fit Super Show Men's Physique Competition
- 2014 – Crossfit Team Shootout

Facebook: Team Vegan Rhinos - facebook.com/groups/TeamVeganRhinos/

Twitter: @rasskt

Instagram: rasskt

Born and raised in Panama City, Panama, Roger was very physically active from an early age. He played soccer and baseball in his primary years and basketball throughout high school.

At the age of twenty-four, during a conversation with his friend Rapha, the topic of veganism came up. Rapha told Roger that if he wanted to really know about the lifestyle, he needed to get educated. He gave him the book, *Mucusless Diet Healing System,* by Arnold Erhet. Roger read the book, but still wasn't completely convinced about the whole vegan thing.

A month later, Roger and his friend traveled to Argentina. There they met some great vegan friends. That experience, along with viewing slaughterhouse videos on the PETA (People for the Ethical Treatment of Animals) website, was instrumental in his decision to switch to a vegan lifestyle, immediately.

Roger now trains for bodybuilding, a journey he began in 2008. His goals are to build the best physique possible on a plant-based diet, and to promote veganism in the state of Texas where he resides. He weight trains six days per week, trains CrossFit twice a week, and is constantly researching ways to improve his workouts. He follows a three split routine with focus on training legs, heavy lifting in general, and a high raw vegan diet consisting of about 3,000 calories daily. In the summer of 2014, Roger joined his mentor, Robert Cheeke, in his first physique competition in Austin, TX.

Amber Sperling

Birth year: 1989

Became plant-based: 2012

Height: 5' 8"

Weight: 155 pounds

Sport: CrossFit

Athletic highlights:

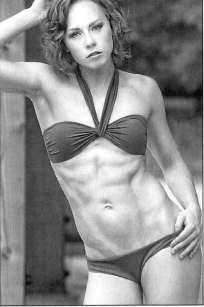

Photo by Rafid Khan

- May 11, 2013 – 11th of 15 – Tall Bikini Class B – NPC Powerhouse Pro Am Classic
- May 25, 2013 – 7th of 8 – Tall Bikini Class D – Mike Vruggink's NPC Grand Rapids Championships
- January 11, 2014 – 2nd of 9 (Medium weight division) – Plymouth CrossFit Yeti Competition
- January 26, 2014 – 26th of 102 Teams – Oakland County Cross-Fit, Chicks and Dicks - Partner Competition (w/Ricky Middlebrook)
- July 26, 2014 – 2nd Place – Naturally Fit Super Show CrossFit Competition

Facebook: facebook.com/herbivorewellness

Twitter: @ambersperling

Amber is a business professional, fitness fanatic, bikini competitor turned cross fitter, green belt in karate-do, and is passionate about sharing the health benefits of a plant-based diet with others. She is driven by results and motivated by challenges. In all factors of her life, she consistently drives herself to perform above the standard. She takes great pleasure in her work, obsesses over details, and is on an endless quest for success. She conditions her body with strength and endurance training. She also trains in Matsubayashi-Ryu Karate-Do, for her mind, body, and soul. Her boyfriend, Richard, has been a large influence in her life; together they foster a healthy lifestyle. As a vegan athlete, Amber sees it as her mission to break stereotypes and be an example for others, on how to build a healthy, lean, and muscular body while sustaining a plant-based diet.

Since adopting a plant-based diet, she has felt energized, healthy, and can't remember the last time she was sick. "Fueling your body properly, allows you to perform at your full potential," she said. She noticed a difference in her outlook on life, she feels happier, more ambitious, and healthy. "When you eat a clean plant-based diet you are in sync with your body, and can identify problems in your nutrition immediately," she added. Amber no longer suffers from uncomfortable side effects that food may ward such as bloating, indigestion, or upset stomach. "You don't have to take a pill to fix these problems. Rethink what you are putting in your body, eat to perform, and don't live to eat," she said. One thing her journey has taught her is that it's never too late to take control of your life!

Korin Sutton

Birth year: 1985

Became plant-based: 2013

Height: 5' 10"

Weight: 185 pounds

Sport: Bodybuilding, Stand-up Paddle Boarding "SUP", Tennis, Racquet Ball, and Competitive Shooting

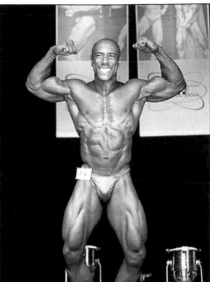

Photo by Tony Wilder

Athletic highlights:

- 2013 – 1st Overall Novice, 2nd Men's Open – ANBF Boca Brick House (First Competition)

- 2013 – 1st Overall Novice, 2nd Men's Open Middle Weight – NPC Ruby Championship

- 2013 – 3rd Men's Open Heavy Weight – DFAC Florida State Natural

- 2013 – 5th Men's Middle Weight – NGA American National Championships

- 2013 – 1st Men's Open Middle Weight – NPC Florida Gold Cup Classic

- 2013 – 2nd Men's Open – ANBF Natural Conch Republic and Pro All Star Challenge

- 2014 – 1st "PRO CARD" Men's Open Division ANBF Boca Brick House Classic

- 2014 – 1st Open Men's Bodybuilding, 1st Overall Men Bodybuilding "PRO CARD" NGA Pro Abraham Championships

- 2014 – 1st Place Light Heavyweight – INBF Naturally Fit Super Show

Website: bodyhdfitness.com

Facebook: facebook.com/korin.sutton

Twitter: @KorinSutton

Instagram: korinsutton

Ever since Korin became vegan, he says it is the best decision he has ever made. He has always been a very active person, especially in the gym. "Living on a plant-based diet is the most rewarding and most compassionate lifestyle to live," he said. He is a proud vegan bodybuilder and feels honored to compete and stand for animal rights. By following a plant-based diet, he is in the best shape of his life and he is not supporting the killing of another animal. "There are no negative effects of living a plant-based lifestyle, just positive benefits," he said. Korin is an ISSA Certified Sport Nutritionist and Fitness Trainer, Mad Dogg Athletics Certified SPIN Instructor, and has an A.A. in Exercise Science. As a walking example of a successful plant-based athlete, this is the best Korin has ever felt physically and mentally.

Thomas Tadlock

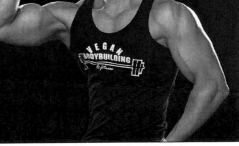

Birth year: 1976

Became plant-based: 2011

Height: 5' 11"

Weight: 180 to 205 pounds depending on athletic focus

Website:
VeganMuscleBook.com

Facebook: facebook.com/ThomasTadlock

Twitter: @thomastadlock

Photo by Melissa Schwartz - theveganrevolution.net

Thomas has been recognized as one of the top five trainers in the USA, with his first personal training company, winning the "Best of Award" six years in a row, and his second company becoming the largest indoor fitness boot camp in Orange County, CA. He was MTV's 2003 Hottest Body winner, and is currently the host of one of the top fitness podcasts on the Internet, the Vegan Body Revolution Show.

Thomas has successfully led trainings for thousands of individuals, organizations, and entrepreneurs, nationwide, including professional recording artists, models, and entrepreneurs. He is a master trainer for three different fitness companies and has been featured on multiple fitness DVDs. He has been sought after and has worked with top personal trainers of celebrities like Britney Spears and professional sports teams including the Los Angeles Angels of Anaheim. He holds a Master's Degree in Exercise Science & Health Promotion and eight national fitness certifications.

Thomas is an inventor and fitness patent holder, creating the world's first patented muscle tempo training system. He is an internationally recognized trainer educator, and has authored the weight loss programs for the fitness equipment company behind the hit TV show, "The Biggest Loser."

He is a professional speaker who has shared the stage with the likes of Dr. John Gray, author of the best-selling book *Men are from Mars, Women are from Venus*, Health Gurus David Wolfe, JJ Virgin, Rob Sugar, and many more. Thomas has successfully cracked the code on how to build muscle and lose body fat on a 100 percent plant-based diet and has a mission to help everyone achieve their ultimate dream bodies.

Dani Taylor

Birth year: 1986

Became plant-based: 2003

Height: 5' 7"

Weight: 135 pounds

Sports: Bodybuilding, Figure Competitor

Athletic highlights:

- 2014 – 2nd Place in Debut, 4th Place in Novice, 3rd Place in Open OCB – Spirit of America

- 2014 – 1st place, INBF Naturally Fit Super Show

Photo by James Scarpetta

- Coached many successful vegan physique athletes

Website: VeganProteins.com

Facebook: facebook.com/VeganProteins

Twitter: @VeganProteins @PlantBuilt

Instagram: VeganProteins

Growing up as an overweight vegetarian, Dani was very surprised when she lost thirty pounds fairly quickly after turning to veganism for ethical reasons at the age of seventeen. This weight loss inspired to her to begin working out and eating better and she continued to drop a total of 80 pounds and get down to a healthy weight for the first time in her life. When she became curious about weightlifting to build muscle in 2007, no trainer would work with her, claiming, "You won't get enough protein to build muscle on a vegan diet." After meeting Robert Cheeke at the Boston Vegetarian Festival in 2007, she became inspired to make it happen. She took to training herself and learning as much as she could about plant-based athletic nutrition. She has gone on to become a personal trainer and a coach to many successful vegan physique competitors, as well as successfully competing in figure competitions herself. Together, Dani and her fiancé, Giacomo Marchese, founded Team PlantBuilt, the competitive vegan muscle team. She plans on continuing to help disprove the myths about what is possible on a fully plant-based diet, and help others to do the same.

Marcella Torres

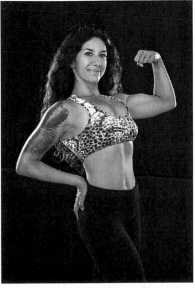

Birth year: 1981

Became plant-based: 2000

Height: 5' 2"

Weight: 120 pounds

Sport: Bodybuilding, Dance

Athletic highlights:

- 2013 – 2nd Place Women's Body-building – Naturally Fit Super Show

Website: VeganMuscleandFitness.com

Facebook: facebook.com/veganmuscle

Photo by Melissa Schwartz - theveganrevolution.net

Marcella, formerly a professional mathematician, is now a competitive vegan bodybuilder, professional dancer, coauthor of *The Vegan Muscle & Fitness Guide to Bodybuilding Competitions*, coauthor of the Vegan Muscle & Fitness blog, and co-owner of plant-based personal training studio Root Force Personal Training in Richmond, VA with husband Derek Tresize. She became vegan for ethical reasons in 2001 after a friend lent her a copy of *Diet for a New America* but soon discovered that vastly improved health was a spectacular fringe benefit of this lifestyle choice! Formerly obese, Marcella quickly shed the excess weight and has been training since 2007, seeing excellent gains in strength and muscle on a plant-based diet. She is also mother to a healthy, happy vegan toddler and attributes his incredible compassion (and energy) to their family's diet as well.

Derek Tresize

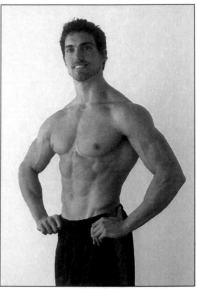

Birth year: 1987

Became plant-based: 2007

Height: 5' 11"

Weight: 190 pounds

Sport: Bodybuilding

Athletic highlights:

- 2012 – Men's Tall Division Champion – OCB Bodysculpt Open
- 2013 – Light Heavyweight Champion – Naturally Fit Super Show

Photo by Kimberly Frost

- 2014 – Men's Physique Champion – Naturally Fit Super Show

Website: VeganMuscleandFitness.com

Facebook: facebook.com/veganmuscle

Twitter: @veganmuscle

Instagram: veganmuscleandfitness

Derek is a competitive vegan bodybuilder residing in Richmond, VA. He holds a Bachelor of Science degree in Biology, is a personal trainer through the American Council on Exercise, has a certificate in Plant-Based Nutrition through Cornell University, and is coauthor of *The Vegan Muscle & Fitness Guide to Bodybuilding Competitions*, and the website VeganMuscleAndFitness.com. Derek has followed a plant-based diet since 2007 and promotes it to his clients and in the fitness and bodybuilding communities as the best means to fitness and long-term health. He is also a three-time bodybuilding/physique champion, in three different divisions.

Will Tucker

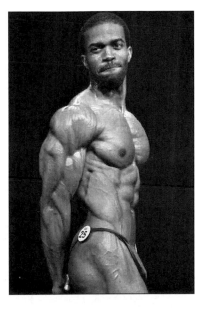

Birth year: 1970

Became plant-based: 2011

Height: 5' 7"

Weight: 152 pounds

Sport: Bodybuilding

Athletic highlights:

- 2009 – 3rd Place – NPC Arizona Natural Bodybuilding Contest
- 2010 – 2nd Place – OCB Arizona Natural Bodybuilding Contest
- 2011 – 1st Place Men's Open Short – OCB Arizona Natural Bodybuilding Contest
- 2011 – 1st Place Master's 40+ – OCB Arizona Natural Bodybuilding Contest
- 2011 – Master's Overall Champion, *Pro Card Awarded – OCB Arizona Natural Bodybuilding Contest
- 2013 – 4th Place Light Heavyweight – IFPA Master's Pro Cup St. Louis
- 2013 – 3rd Place Open Lightweight – Naturally Fit Supershow
- 2013 – 1st Place Masters 40+ – Naturally Fit Supershow
- 2013 – Master's Overall Champion – Naturally Fit Super Show
- 2014 – 2nd Place, Masters 40+ – Naturally Fit Super Show

Website: fitnessbywill.com

Facebook: facebook.com/pages/The-Freakin-Vegan-IFPA-Pro-Bodybuilder/221421887887702

Twitter: @thefreakinvegan

Being raised in East St. Louis, IL, meat was served at every meal for Will. He would unconsciously consume massive amounts of animal products without thinking about it. "It was the normal thing to do," he said. In fact, if there was no meat available with a meal it seemed unnatural. Little did he know that as he grew older his mentality would take a monumental shift. During the summer of 1991 he read the book, *How To Not Eat Pork,* by Shahrazad Ali. This book convinced him to stop eating pork cold turkey. Following that, in the year 2000, he gave up red meat almost entirely. He would occasionally have a burger, but it was rarely. His meat preferences were now down to chicken, fish, and turkey. Fast-forward to Thanksgiving 2006 and the major shift began.

After celebrating a "traditional" Thanksgiving with friends he returned home and found himself watching a National Geographic documentary about animals being born. There was something about that program that awakened his spiritual subconscious and made him realize that he was eating a living, breathing creature much like himself. Immediately, he threw out all leftovers from dinner, cleared his refrigerator of all meat products and has not consumed meat since. He stopped drinking milk at the same time, and his only remaining vices were eggs and cheese. He was a vegetarian, but in 2011, he decided to eliminate the remaining animal products from his life and has never looked back. "Becoming vegan is the best decision I have ever made!" he exclaims. "As a professional natural bodybuilder, I truly believe this gives me an edge over the typical 'meat-head' athlete because my nutritional profile is chock-full of healthy, delicious food that is also cruelty-free," he added.

Torre Washington

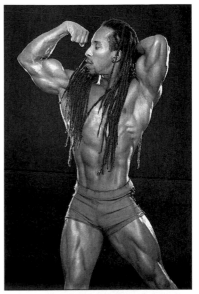

Birth year: 1974

Became plant-based: 1998 (vegetarian since birth)

Height: 5' 7"

Weight: 170 pounds

Sport: Bodybuilding

Athletic Highlights:

- 2009 – 3rd Place – SNBF
- 2009 – 1st Place – SNBF
- 2011 – 3rd Place – SNBF (Pro)
- 2011 – 3rd Place – Musclemania
- 2012 – 3rd Place – SNBF (Pro)
- 2012 – 3rd Place – IFPA (Pro)
- 2012 – 2nd Place – Musclemania
- 2013 – 1st Place – IFPA (Pro)
- 2013 – 2nd Place – SNBF (Pro)
- 2013 – 1st Place – Musclemania
- 2013 – 1st Place (Overall) – INBF
- 2013 – 1st Place (Nationally Qualified) – NPC State

Photo by Melissa Schwartz - theveganrevolution.net

Website: thaveganread.com

Facebook: facebook.com/ThaVeganDread

Twitter: @thavegandread

Torre, "Tha Vegan Dread," is a champion bodybuilder, who has mystified many spectators and judges alike with his aesthetic physique. In the fitness world, largely based on the notion that animal protein is the best and only source of quality protein, Torre has emerged as a champion bodybuilder, shattering that outdated belief system.

Tha Vegan Dreads' goal is to inspire people whether they follow a plant-based diet or not, to adopt a lifestyle free of restrictions that lead to an abnormal way of thinking about one's ability to achieve their dreams, whether fitness or otherwise. His premise is to encourage people to engineer a healthy balanced life where one can enjoy the freedoms they so desire. The Lion and the Leaf of his brand logo represent the courage and strength coupled with the compassion for species of all kinds. Simply put, "balance," is the message he aims to convey.

Torre has seen his share of setbacks on and off the stage but realizes that with hard work and determination, anything is possible if you set your mind to it. His current goals are to continue spreading the message that living an Ital (plant-based) way of life can do a lot of good for the world, by sharing his story and physique as a positive example for all.

Even with five bodybuilding championship wins, Torre realizes there is more work to be done in creating a legacy. As he loves to say, "Let's Get It!"

Alicia Ziegler

Birth year: 1981

Became plant-based: 1994

Height: 5' 4"

Weight: 120 pounds off-season, 114 pounds in-season

Sport: Competitive bikini competitions, half marathons, and 15Ks are most recent; climbing Mt. Fuji and Kilimanjaro soon!

Athletic highlights:

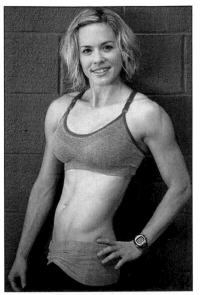

Photo by Michael Worth

- Winning her very first contest in Las Vegas at the Miss Bikini America Show

Facebook: facebook.com/ActressZiegler

Twitter: @AliciaZiegler

Alicia was born in Oxnard, CA. A life-long Southern California girl, she took an interest in entertainment and fitness at a very young age, gaining a position on both the crew team and as cheerleader while studying in college. Graduating in just three years from Chapman University with a B.F.A. in film production, Alicia also obtained her Masters of Science in Health and Nutrition Education from Hawthorn University to round out her two favorite fields.

Alicia's penchant for challenge brought her to enter the Los Angeles Marathon on one week's notice and ultimately completing the event in less than five hours. Her introduction to the benefits of weight training came while preparing for the Lavaman Triathlon when she injured her rotator cuff in her shoulder. Weight training became her therapy and soon an enormous part of her athletic life. It was within a year of her newfound rehabilitation that she found herself being approached about competing in a fitness show. "Nothing is impossible to a willing heart," Alicia notes as one of her favorite motivational quotes. Not one to turn down a healthy test, Alicia found herself three months later competing and ultimately winning the MuscleMania Miss Bikini Contest in Las Vegas. Having taken on the challenge with no knowledge or understanding of competition preparation, Alicia realized her instincts were ripe for this fitness vocation.

She followed up with the Avon 3-Day Breast Cancer Walk as well as taking on youth counselor duties at Camp Del Corazon for children with heart disease. Her acting roles began to broaden into more fitness oriented characters including tennis players, roller derby, and even surfing in the feature film *A Beautiful Wave*. Now experienced in CrossFit training, spin, and even some martial arts, Alicia is preparing for her next fitness competition. With a steady acting career that includes a starring role in the adventure film "Jurassic Attack," Alicia's future goals of combining both her entertainment and fitness loves in her new company Mox-Z Fitness are now, like her initial strength competitions, just one focused effort away for this young ambitious contender!

– CHAPTER 12 –

Epic Plant-Based Athlete Photo Collage

> *"Our deepest fear is not that we are inadequate. Our deepest fear is that we are powerful beyond measure. It is our light, not our darkness that most frightens us. You playing small does not serve the world. There is nothing enlightened about shrinking so that other people won't feel insecure around you. We are all meant to shine, as children do. It's not just in some of us; it's in everyone. And as we let our own light shine, we unconsciously give other people permission to do the same. As we are liberated from our own fear, our presence automatically liberates others."*
>
> — Marianne Williamson

For the past decade I have toured all over North America and beyond, and have met countless plant-based athletes along the way. I have been a guest speaker at festivals, colleges, universities, libraries, conventions, bookstores, grocery stores, and in many other settings including cruise ships, weekend emersion programs and retreats. I have attended health and fitness events from coast to coast and have been on a book tour with *Vegan Bodybuilding & Fitness* for the past four years. During that time, I have met many wonderful people who live a compassionate plant-based fitness lifestyle. I enthusiastically share some of their photos with you in this chapter. From the motivational and inspirational images, to the silly and adventurous ones, this is what we call an epic plant-based athlete photo collage.

I hope these images inspire you to want to follow *your* passion and make it happen! Ready, set, FLEX!

Shred It!

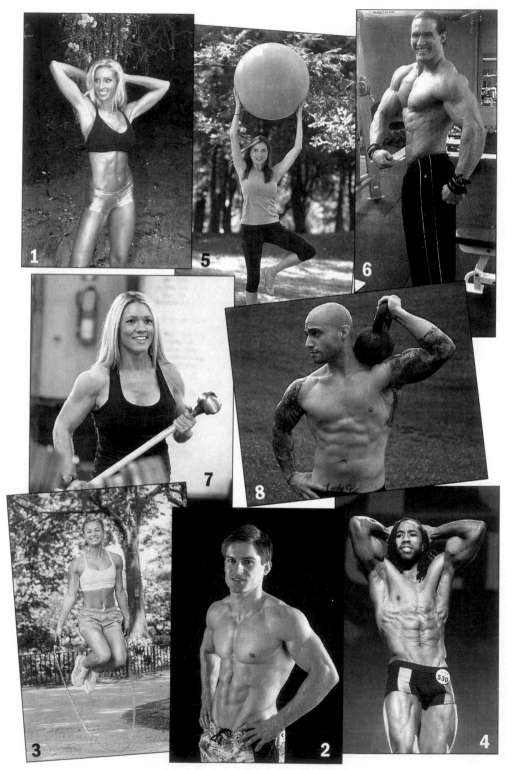

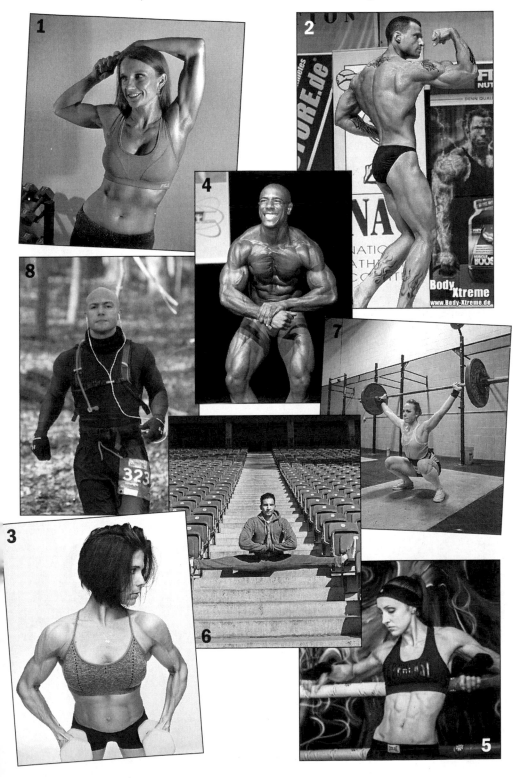

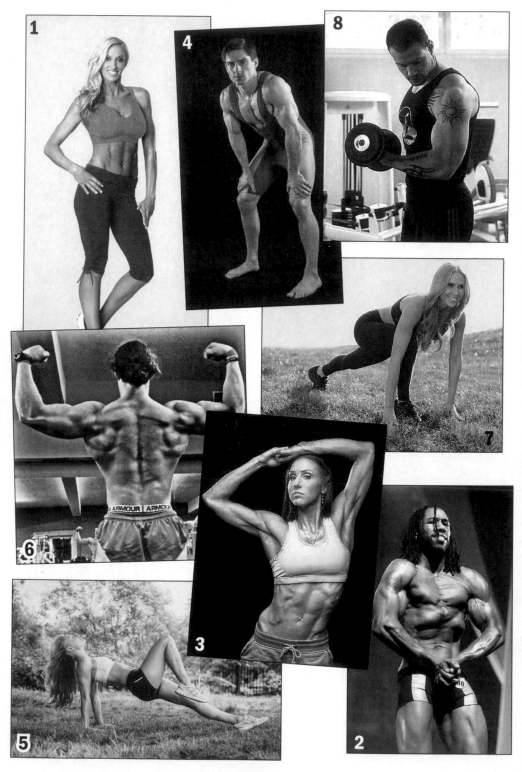

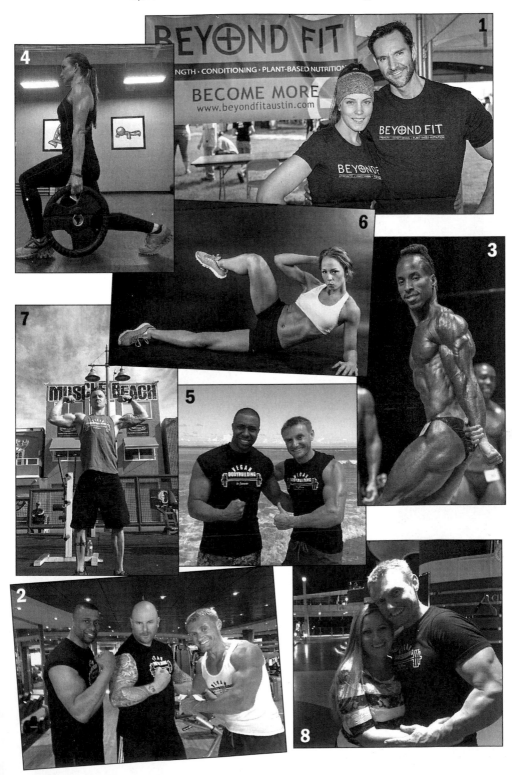

Shred It!

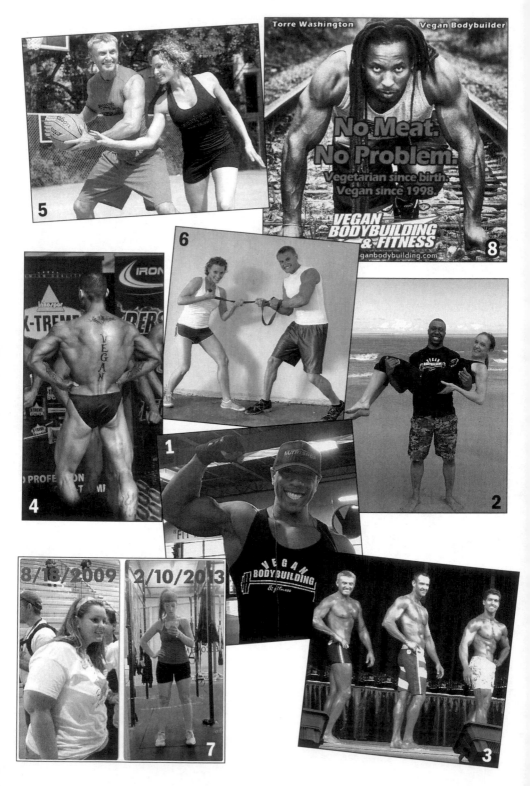

Collage Photo Credits

Page 320:
1. Monica Parodi – Photo by Jason Ellis
2. Tobias Klingl – Photo by Falko Werner - picture4u.de
3. Lauren Goebel – Photo by Amber Gress
4. Richard Campbell – Photo by David Ford
5. Elena Kulakovska
6. Ryan Nelson
7. Tiffany Burich – Photo by M-Magee Photography
8. Joel Rosario

Page 321:
1. Jojo Hulett – Photo by Mitch Espat
2. Arvid Beck – Photo by BodyXtreme.de
3. Melissa Hauser – Photo by Sarah Lechner - sarahreneephoto.zenfolio.com
4. Korin Sutton – Photo by Tony Wilder
5. Simone Collins
6. Attila Hildmann – Photo by Sandra Czerny
7. Amber Sperling
8. Joel Rosario

Page 322:
1. Monica Parodi – Photo by Todd Vitti
2. Richard Campbell – Photo by David Ford
3. Simone Collins – Photo by Mark Hillyer Photography - markhillyer.com.au
4. Tobias Klingl – Photo by Falko Werner -picture4u.de
5. Lauren Goebel – Photo by Amber Gress
6. Ryan Nelson
7. Marzia Prince – Photo by Wade Livingston - wadelivingston.com
8. Arvid Beck – Photo by Bettina Matic - Moderne Fotografie

Page 323:
1. Tricia Kelly and Chad Byers – Photo by Heather Schramm - Austin Vivid Photography
2. Roger Smith, Chris Rowe, and Robert Cheeke
3. Torre Washington – Photo by Raymond Moore
4. Jojo Hulett
5. Roger Smith and Robert Cheeke
6. Amber Sperling – Photo by Jason Bennett Photography Out of the Box
7. Ed Bauer
8. Karen Oxley and Robert Cheeke

Page 324:
1. Korin Sutton
2. Roger Smith and Jojo Hulett – Photo by Robert Cheeke
3. Robert Cheeke, Chad Byers, and Derek Tresize – Photo by Tricia Kelly
4. Arvid Beck – Photo by Marco Rockel (MaRoPhoto/Gelsenkirchen, Germany)
5. Robert Cheeke and Mindy Collette – Photo by Brenda Carey
6. Mindy Collette and Robert Cheeke – Photo by Austin Barbisch
7. Tricia Kelly
8. Torre Washington – Photo by Ira Lewis - Text graphics by Richard Watts

– CHAPTER 13 –

Resources

> *"The greater the loyalty of a group toward the group, the greater is the motivation among the members to achieve the goals of the group, and the greater the probability that the group will achieve its goals."*
>
> — Rensis Likert

Use the following resources to learn more, get connected, network with others, and continue to be a valuable part of the growing plant-based community. This is just a sample of what is available on the Internet. Refer to the www.veganbodybuilding.com Resources Page, or your own online searches for additional helpful resources.

Plant-Based Personal Trainer Directory

I do not have a personal relationship with every trainer listed, nor do I know their level of expertise or quality of work. In addition to the personal trainers I do know, I completed online searches to come up with this list to save you time. For ease of locating someone near you, you will find their location and their website listed below, just as they publicly share that information on their public social media pages and websites. Many of these trainers offer online personal training in addition to in-person one-on-one or group personal training classes and bootcamps.

There are more than seventy-five plant-based personal trainers from around the world listed below for you to reference. If you are seeking the help of a personal trainer, you have a wide variety of experts to choose from. I have included their websites to save you an extra step in trying to find them online, but please note that some websites change over time. At the time of this printing all websites and social media pages listed are accurate and active links. If for some reason a link is no longer active, simply search the individual by name. The trainers are listed alphabetically by last name.

Ellen Abraham (Greenfield, MA) – theveganloveproject.com

Austin Barbisch (Austin, TX) – solidpt.com

Eric Bartholomae (San Diego, CA) – facebook.com/XVeganstraightedgeX

Ed Bauer (San Francisco, CA) – edbauerfit.com

Rachel Bents (St. Paul, MN) – twitter.com/EnjoyWellnessMN

Alli Breen (Portland, OR) – theallib.com

Melissa Brey (Irvine, CA) – facebook.com/melissa.brey.948?fref=ts

Tiffany Burich (Ft. Lauderdale, FL) – NoExcusesFitness.org

Chad Byers (Austin, TX) – beyondfitaustin.com

Richard Campbell (Toronto, ON Canada) – livityfitness.com

Melissa Carr (Chicago, IL) – facebook.com/BodifiedbyMel

Kappel Clarke (Los Angeles, CA) – facebook.com/kappel.clarke?fref=ts

Mindy Collette (New York City, NY) – mindyvegan.com

Gemma Cooke (Bristol, UK) – gemmacpt.com

Jayna Davis (Pennsylvania) – rawfitmama.blogspot.com

Kyle den Bak (Ottawa, ON Canada) – twitter.com/kdenBak

Paola Deocampo (Pasadena, CA) – paolasvoice.tumblr.com

Erin Fergus (Greer, SC) – facebook.com/girlybodybuilder

Amanda Fisher (Queensland, Australia) – banginbodz.com

David Fisher (Bedford, UK) – davidjfisher.wordpress.com

Dan Fivey (Cheltenham, UK) – danfiveypersonaltraining.co.uk

Alexandra Gray (Arizona) – twitter.com/_Alexandrasgray

Scott Green (Los Angeles, CA) – facebook.com/scott.green.522?fref=ts

Ben Greene (Seattle, WA) – greenemultisport.com

Christine Heggestad (Kansas City, MO) – facebook.com/
    LivingCleanWithChristine/info

Jon Hinds (Chicago, IL) – jonnyhinds.blogspot.com

Lucy Howlett (Brighton, UK) – liftpersonal-training.co.uk

Hope Hughes (Georgia) – veganrenegade.com

Matthew Hughes (Banbury, UK) – mybodybuildingtrip.wordpress.com

Karina Inkster (Vancouver, BC Canada) – karinainkster.com

Neda Iranpour (San Diego, CA) – lightenupwithneda.com

Ellen Jaffe Jones (Holmes Beach, FL) – vegcoach.com
Harley Johnstone (Australia) – durianrider.com
Tricia Kelly (Austin, TX) – beyondfitaustin.com
Shane Lamers (Scottsdale, AZ) – facebook.com/scottsdalepersonaltrainer
Christina Leid (New Orleans, LA) – inspirehealthmag.com
Mike Mahler (Las Vegas, NV) – mikemahler.com
Jehina Malik (Brooklyn, NY) – facebook.com/jehina.malik.5
Ashli McKee (Austin, TX) – about.me/ashli
Miranda McPherson (Calgary, AB Canada) – miranda-mcpherson.com
Lani Meulrath (California) – lanimuelrath.com
Jennifer Moore (Memphis, TN) – vegwell.com
Christy Morgan (Austin, TX) – theblissfulchef.com
Justin Morgan (Dayton, OH) – facebook.com/justin.morgan.9659?fref=ts
Jason Morris (Portland, OR) – ironethospdx.com
Ryan Nelson (Minneapolis, MN) – alphafitnessmn.com
Mary Nguyen (Paris, France) – evolvewithfitmarypt.webs.com
Kevin Park (Victoria, BC Canada) – rewildyourbody.com/30dayprogram/
Charles Parker (Ft. Lauderdale, FL) – cp3nutrifit.com
Nick Patenaude (Victoria, BC Canada) – tri-nick.ca
Juan Perez (Brentwood, CA) – twitter.com/JuanP_training
John Pierre (Boulder, CO) – johnpierre.com
Fawn Porter (Sydney, Australia) – facebook.com/fawn.porter.1?fref=ts
Mike Portman (San Francisco, CA) – portmancoaching.com
Marzia Prince (Dallas, TX) – MarziaPrince.com
Yolanda Presswood (Los Angeles, CA) – pwdfitness.com
Meg Ramsey (Nocona, TX) – megafitthoughts.blogspot.com
Amanda Riester (Los Angeles, CA) – facebook.com/VeganAthlete
Victor Rivera (Los Angeles, CA) – veganpowertraining.wordpress.com
Sara Russert (Seattle, WA) – facebook.com/veganpowerhousephysiques
Taylor Ryan (Charleston, SC) – liftingrevolution.com
Melike Sayman (Madrid, Spain) – twitter.com/RunningCinnamon
Max Seabrook (London, England) – facebook.com/maxseabrook? fref=tl_
    fr_box
Christa Shelton (Los Angeles, CA) – vegginoutwithchrista.com
Scott Shetler (Atlanta, GA) – plantbasedperformance.org
Shanique Small (Toronto, ON Canada) – twitter.com/shaniqueolivia
Mary Stella Stabinsky (Plains, PA) – facebook.com/mary.stabinsky
Petra Axlund Stegman (Stockholm, Sweden) – twitter.com/petraaxlund

Thomas Tadlock (Austin, TX) – thomastadlock.com
Luke Tan (Melbourne, Australia) – evolvedgeneration.com
Dani Taylor (Haverhill, MA) – facebook.com/veganpowerhousephysiques
Jenn Thrift (Colorado) – jennthrift.com
Marcella Torres (Richmond, VA) – veganmuscleandfitness.com
Derek Tresize (Richmond, VA) – veganmuscleandfitnesss.com
Will Tucker (Gilbert, AZ) – bodyfusion.com
Damon Valley (Los Angeles, CA) – damonvalley.tumblr.com
Kim Waldauer (Los Angeles, CA) – habitfitnessla.com
Koya Webb (Los Angeles, CA) – koyawebb.com
Carli Wheatley Goss (London, England) – twitter.com/CarliGoss
Jana Yowell (Sugar Land, TX) – runningvegan.com
Hayley Zedel (Victoria, BC Canada) – holistichayley.wordpress.com

Refer to *Vegan Health & Fitness Magazine* for an ongoing, updated directory:
veganhealthandfitnessmag.com/fitness-professionals/
Visit veganbodybuilding.com for additional resources.

Plant-Based Registered Dietitian Directory

Krissy Adams – facebook.com/FitStartsHere.ca
Andy Bellatti – smallbites.andybellatti.com
Barbara Chin – twitter.com/barbarajchin
Joanne Christaldi – twitter.com/jchristaldi76
Brenda Davis – brendadavisrd.com
George Eisman – all-creatures.org/ccp/
Allyson Geshwenter – runninggreen.blogspot.com
Julieanna Hever – plantbaseddietitian.com
Rachael McBride – rachaelmcbride.com/about-rachael.html
Vesanto Melina – nutrispeak.com
Ginny Messina – theveganrd.com
Jack Norris – jacknorrisrd.com
Jeff Novick – jeffnovick.com/RD/Home.html
Jill Nussinow – theveggiequeen.com
Colleen Poling – nutritiontranslator.com
Leslie Riding – twitter.com/LocalVegRD
Valerie Rosser – thevegandietitian.com
Matt Ruscigno – truelovehealth.com
Anya Todd – anyatodd.com

Plant-Based Doctor Directory

Dr. Neal Barnard – pcrm.org

Dr. Linda Carney – drcarney.com

Dr. Garth Davis – thedavisclinic.com

Dr. Caldwell Esselstyn Jr. – heartattackproof.com

Dr. Joel Fuhrman – drfuhrman.com

Dr. Brooke Goldner – VeganMedicalDoctor.com

Dr. Michael Greger – nutritionfacts.org

Dr. Matthew Lederman – transitiontohealth.com

Dr. John McDougall – drmcdougall.com

Dr. Milton Mills – responsibleeatingandliving.com/?page_id=4225

Dr. Baxter Montgomery – drbaxtermontgomery.com

Dr. Pam Popper – wellnessforum.com

Dr. Alona Pulde – transitiontohealth.com

Dr. Dean Ornish – pmri.org/dean_ornish.html

Plant-Based Fitness Websites

badassvegan.com

nomeatathlete.com

plantbuilt.com

veganbodybuilding.com

veganbodybuilding.org

veganhealthandfitnessmagazine.com

veganmuscleandfitness.com

veganproteins.com

Online Plant-Based Athlete Communities

facebook.com/NoMeatAthlete

facebook.com/VeganBodybuildingAndFitness

facebook.com/groups/VeganBodybuildingAndFitness

Books

Basic Course in Vegan and Vegetarian Nutrition – all-creatures.org/ccp/
index.shtml

Engine 2 Diet – engine2diet.com

Forks Over Knives The Cookbook – forksoverknives.com
No Meat Athlete – nomeatathlete.com
The China Study – thechinastudy.com
The Complete Idiot's Guide to Plant-Based Nutrition –
   plantbaseddietitian.com
The Forks Over Knives Plan – forksoverknives.com
The Pillars of Health – johnpierre.com
The Vegan Muscle & Fitness Guide to Bodybuilding Competitions –
   veganmuscleandfitness.com
The World Peace Diet – worldpeacediet.org
Thrive – brendanbrazier.com
Thrive Fitness – brendanbrazier.com
Vegan Bodybuilding & Fitness – veganbodybuilding.com
Whole – thechinastudy.com/whole/about/

Documentaries

Cowspiracy – cowspiracy.com
Earthlings – earthlings.com
Forks Over Knives – forksoverknives.com
Mad Cowboy – madcowboy.com
Peaceable Kingdom: The Journey Home – peaceablekingdomfilm.org
Speciesism – speciesismthemovie.com
Vegucated – getvegucated.com

Podcasts

Mike Mahler's Live Life Aggressively Podcast – mikemahler.com/blog
No Meat Athlete Podcast – nomeatathlete.com
Rich Roll Podcast – richroll.com
Vegan Body Revolution Show – veganbodyrevolution.com

Events

Engine 2 Diet Retreats (Many locations around US) – engine2retreats.com
Farm Sanctuary Hoe Down (Upstate NY and Northern CA) –
   farmsanctuary.org/events
Healthy You Network (Tucson, AZ) – healthyyounetwork.org

Holistic Holiday at Sea, vegan-themed cruise (Caribbean) –
    atasteofhealth.org
New Year, New You Health Fest (Marshall, TX) –
    newyearnewyouhealthfest.com
Vegetarian Summerfest (Johnstown, PA) – vegetariansummerfest.com

Vegetarian Festivals (VegFests)

Today, nearly every major U.S. city has a vegetarian festival (often called a
VegFest) and many major metropolitan cities around the world have some
sort of vegetarian, vegan, or plant-based festival, conference, event, or
meet-up group. Search online for the one nearest you. Some of my personal
favorite events based on the quality of educational presenters, and from my
first-hand experience attending them are listed below:

Boston Vegetarian Food Festival (Boston, MA) – bostonveg.org/foodfest
Central Florida VegFest (Orlando, FL) – cfvegfest.org
Chicago Vegan Mania (Chicago, IL) – chicagoveganmania.com
DC VegFest (District of Columbia) – dcvegfest.com
New Orleans VegFest (New Orleans, LA) – nolaveggiefest.com
Portland VegFest (Portland, OR) – nwveg.org/vegfest
Tampa VegFest (Tampa, FL) – tampavegfest.org
Texas VegFest (Austin, TX) – texasvegfest.com
Toronto Vegetarian Food Festival (Toronto, ON) – festival.veg.ca
WorldFest (Los Angeles, CA) – worldfestevents.com
World Vegetarian Day Festival (San Francisco, CA) – worldvegfestival.com
There are plenty of other VegFests around the world, including many in
    Europe and Australia.
Some links that provide comprehensive lists of vegetarian/vegan/plant-
    based and health-themed events include the following:
It's Easy Being Vegan – itseasybeingvegan.com/resources/vegan-and-
    vegetarian-festivals-events-and-conferences/
The Vegan Voice – theveganvoice.org/events/
Veggie Focus – veggiefocus.com/blog/vegetarian-vegan-festivals-around-
    the-world/

For other meet-ups and events, especially in your region, look to social media
websites that often have geographical interest-themed events easily search-
able on platforms such as Facebook, Twitter, Pintrest, and MeetUp.com.

Sources

Page ix: http://shrp.rutgers.edu/dept/nutr/INI/health/documents/Plant-BasedDiet.pdf

Page 21: http://www.mckinley.illinois.edu/handouts/macronutrients.htm

Page 22: http://nutritionfacts.org/video/do-vegetarians-get-enough-protein/

Page 25: http://www.health.harvard.edu/blog/vitamin-b12-deficiency-can-be-sneaky-harmful-201301105780

Page 26: http://nutritionfacts.org/2011/08/30/3964/

Page 27: http://www.hsph.harvard.edu/nutritionsource/vitamin-d/

Page 50: http://nutritionfacts.org/video/antioxidant-power-of-plant-foods-versus-animal-foods/

– CHAPTER 14 –

Bonus Reading

> *"Anyone who stops learning is old, whether twenty or eighty.*
> *Anyone who keeps learning stays young.*
> *The greatest thing you can do is keep your mind young."*
>
> — Mark Twain

Lucky you! I decided to include some bonus material about why these health, fitness, and environmental issues are so important to so many people that they are covered in hundreds of other books.

What you can do to make a difference

Steps you can take to encourage those around you to adopt a plant-based diet, to lead by example, and shine as a plant-based athlete include:

- Start by shopping for, buying, and consuming plant-based foods right away.

- Educate yourself on the benefits of eating a plant-based diet and work to educate others in your community.

- Go through your pantry, cupboards, refrigerator, and other places you store food in your home and remove all the processed and animal-based foods. Perhaps donate them to a homeless shelter or food bank so they can be of some use rather than just thrown away. Though they provide low nutritional yield, for many who are struggling to find food, something might be better than nothing.

- Grow your own food, even if just one or two plants in a pot by the window or on a deck or patio.

- If you have a family, prepare meals together and educate them on the benefits of a plant-based diet as well as the health risks of consuming animal-based and process foods.

- Prepare your best-tasting and most popular plant-based meals and share them with family, co-workers, teammates, and friends.

- Join a community garden where you can trade work for land or lease space to grow your own food. Cultivate food with your family so they can see where real food comes from, learn how it grows, and appreciate the system from planting to harvest.

- Read books and watch films about the topic of plant-based nutrition. There are numerous, powerful books and videos that are widely accessible all over the world. There are plenty of free websites and resources listed in this book.

- Join a local group, community, or meet-up in your area. There are many vegetarian networks in most major cities in the U.S. and in large cities around the world. Being part of a community can help strengthen desire to share this message with others, while also having a support network as you make new friends and learn from others.

- Be compassionate and understanding when interacting with others who do not see things from your perspective. Practice explaining your lifestyle simply, as Einstein suggested in his famous quote, "If you can't explain it simply, you don't understand it well enough." The better you understand your own viewpoints, the simpler and clearer your explanations and reasoning are likely to be.

Helpful accessible resources to get you started on a healthy plant-based diet today

- T. Colin Campbell Foundation – tcolincampbell.org
- Chef AJ – eatunprocessed.com
- Engine 2 Diet – engine2diet.com
- Dr. Caldwell Esselstyn, Jr. M.D. – heartattackproof.com
- Forks Over Knives – forksoverknives.com
- Dr. John McDougall – drmcdougall.com
- Jeff Novick – jeffnovick.com

- Nutrition Facts – nutritionfacts.org
- Physicians Committee for Responsible Medicine (PCRM) – pcrm.org
- John Pierre – johnpierre.com

Summary

A plant-based diet better serves our health, our environment and our world. It also perfectly complements our athletic endeavors, providing us with the optimal fuel and recovery nutrition to excel in sports. What many of us have suspected all along, happens to be true—a plant-based diet is our best defense against our most prevalent fatal diseases, and can even reverse some diseases and many health complaints, such as heart disease, high cholesterol and obesity. Not only does a plant-based diet reduce our risk of disease, it gives us more control over our health destiny, and helps us save the planet. Nutritionally, it provides us with energy and endurance and helps us recover from exercise efficiently, and provides the building blocks to repair muscle tissues and excel in our athletic pursuits. Environmentally, it changes the world for the better by using fewer resources. It is also a compassionate way to eat and live to respect all life on Earth.

I hope this book will become a blueprint for you to follow to achieve your athletic goals fueled by plants alone. Wishing you all the very best in health and fitness.

Follow *Your* Heart

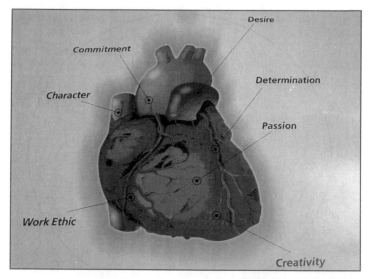

Photo by Robert Cheeke

Acknowledgments

First and foremost, I would like to thank my parents for supporting all of my athletic, academic, professional, and entrepreneurial endeavors over the years. As far back as I can remember, I've been driven to achieve high levels of success in all four realms, and my parents supported and encouraged me around every turn. Mom and Dad, I still have a long way to go to get where I'm going, but I am on my way because of your belief that someday I would find peace and happiness in my pursuit of childhood dreams. Thanks, Mom and Dad. I hope I have made you proud.

I would also like to thank my older sister, Tanya, who introduced me to the vegan lifestyle back in the mid-'90s. It was that specific change in my life nearly two decades ago that ultimately led to this book today. Tanya, you continue to inspire me and you are a great role model for many. I am proud of all you have accomplished and I truly am a lucky little brother to have you as a sister.

My partner, Karen, has supported and encouraged me through this entire writing process. Karen, without your support, understanding, patience and feedback, this book would just be another unfinished project on the back burner somewhere. Thank you for helping bring it to life.

I'd like to extend a special thank you to my website designer and manager, Richard. Richard, thank you for hanging with me over the past decade and keeping VeganBodybuilding.com going strong through all the ups and downs. You've been with me since the beginning and you have been the foundation that has held Vegan Bodybuilding & Fitness up for so long. I sincerely appreciate you and all the great work you do for our brand, for the animals, and the vegan community. Additionally I thank Linus Bourque, Dylan Kasprzyk and James Styler for their leadership and management roles with Vegan Bodybuilding & Fitness, specifically within our interactive community.

I want to thank and acknowledge all of the contributors to this book. I have an amazing group of colleagues who contributed bios, recipes, meal plans, photos, case studies, transformation stories, and additional content. I'd like to recognize Austin Barbisch, Ed Bauer, Arvid Beck, Larry Bennett, Sarah Brightly, Tiffany Burich, Chad Byers, Richard Campbell, Brenda Carey, Tess Challis, Mindy Collette, Simone Collins, Lauren Goebel, Edward Goins, Melissa Hauser, Attila Hildmann, JoJo Hulett, Karina Inkster, Tricia Kelly, Tobias Klingl, Elena Kulakovska, Whitney Lauritsen, Aaron MacNeil, Giacomo Marchese, Ryan Nelson, Jennifer Nicol, Karen Oxley, Monica Parodi, Elana Priesman, Marzia Prince, Joel Rosario, Roger Smith, Amber

Sperling, Korin Sutton, Thomas Tadlock, Dani Taylor, Marcella Torres, Derek Tresize, Will Tucker, Torre Washington, and Alicia Ziegler for their contributions.

Thank you to Jody Conners and Gary Asher from Maverick Publications for creating the cover design, managing the layout, and printing this book. We did it again. Thank you Jody and Gary for giving me a shot at another bestseller. I appreciate your ongoing support and I enjoy working with a team from my home state.

I would like to extend a special thank you to my award-winning editor, Karen Reddick, who taught me a lot about patience and staying the course to keep the message in this book consistent throughout. I learned a lot about writing, editing, and about myself during this editing process. Thank you, Karen, for your outstanding guidance and leadership.

To the women who played such a big role in this book, I would like to extend an extra special thank you to Tess Challis, Mindy Collette, and Elena Kulakovska for going above and beyond with their generous contributions to the recipes, exercise demonstrations, and meal plans we featured. You three ladies are awesome! I am grateful for your wonderful additions that enhanced this book.

I would also like to extend an extra special thank you to photographers, Austin Barbisch, Sarah Brightly, and Brenda Carey for capturing the images that define this book. I sincerely appreciate your time, your efforts, and most importantly, your big hearts for your enthusiasm for this project, helping bring it to life. Thank you also to Melissa Schwartz and Donovan Jenkins for all the great photo shoots over the years, which provided dozens of outstanding photos for this book. I appreciate your attention to detail, quality, and your unwavering compassion for animals.

Thank you to everyone who provided a peer review, an endorsement for the book, critical and helpful feedback, support when I needed it, and a listening ear when I brainstormed and shared ideas. I'd even like to thank my hometown credit union for believing in my project and for supplying me with the loan that made it possible for this book to be printed.

I am grateful to all those who came before me and paved the way for me to perform the work I love and live my passion, and for those who have taken the torch and are running with it to bring awareness to the whole-food, plant-based lifestyle in athletics. I am honored to have the opportunity and platform to share this message with the mainstream public. Without your support this message would be dampened. With your support it is heard around the world. I sincerely thank you for believing in me, for believing in yourselves, and for believing there are brighter days ahead for human and nonhuman animals and for this beautiful planet we call home.

Additionally, I want to thank everyone in the Vegan Bodybuilding & Fitness community. I started a website more than a decade ago to share my experiences as I combined a vegan lifestyle with weightlifting. A community of one quickly turned into hundreds and then thousands. Today we are tens of thousands strong on VeganBodybuilding.com and more than a quarter million strong on combined social media sites. I appreciate each of you. Together, we can change the world. As a hero of mine, Howard Lyman, says in the film Cowspiracy, "You MUST change the world!" Group thumbs up!

Thank You!

Thank you so much for reading my book! I sincerely appreciate your support and I truly hope you enjoyed it and felt it was a good use of your time and money. As always, I wish you the very best in health and fitness. Perhaps I'll see you out on the road when I'm on tour.

If you have questions regarding the content of this book or simply want to get in touch, please use the following methods:

First Option: Write me on Twitter via @RobertCheeke

Second Option: Email info@veganbodybuilding.com

Third Option: Join our Vegan Bodybuilding & Fitness Facebook Group and post questions publicly here: facebook.com/groups/ VeganBodybuildingAndFitness. A team of more than 15,000 plant-based athletes resides there to help answer questions from the community

Get Connected!

Please join us on veganbodybuilding.com as well. We run the largest, most comprehensive and most active plant-based athlete communities on the Internet. We would love to feature you, our fellow plant-based athletes, on our website.

Share!

Please share the information you learned in this book with others. Lead by example in your family, in your community, and in your athletic pursuits. Pass this book along or encourage others to pick up their own copy online or at a book tour event.

I hope you've been inspired to pursue meaningful goals in your life. Thank you for giving me a chance to share stories with you. Thank you so much for supporting my brand, Vegan Bodybuilding & Fitness. I thank you for all the outstanding work you do to make a positive difference in the world. Follow your passion and make it happen!

— Robert Cheeke

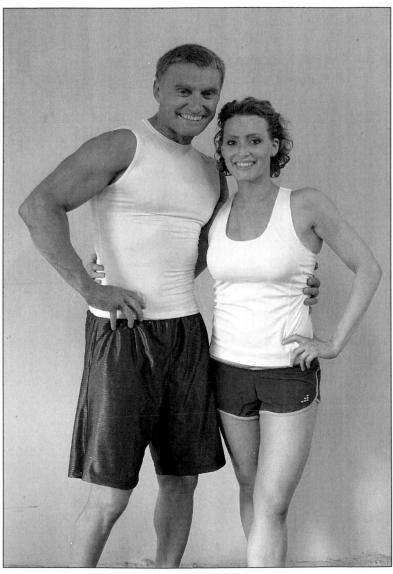

Photo by Austin Barbisch

Connect with our contributors (alphabetical by last name)

Austin Aries – austinhealyaries.com
Austin Barbisch – solidpt.com
Ed Bauer – edbauerfit.com
Gene Baur – farmsanctuary.org
Arvid Beck – arvidbeck.de
Larry Bennett – larrybfit.com
Sarah Brightly – sarahbrightly.com
Tiffany Burich – NoExcusesFitness.org
Grant Butler – oregonlive.com/foodday
Chad Byers – beyondfitaustin.com
Colin Campbell, Ph.D. – nutritionstudies.org
Richard Campbell – livityfitness.com
Brenda Carey – veganhealthandfitnessmag.com
Tess Challis – radianthealth-innerwealth.com
Phil Collen – philcollenpc1.com
Mindy Collette – mindyvegan.com
Simone Collins – simicollins.com
Chloe Coscarelli – chefchloe.com
Mac Danzig – twitter.com/macdanzigmma
Emily Deschanel – twitter.com/emilydeschanel
Mark Devries – speciesismthemovie.com
George Eisman – all-creatures.org/ccp
Caldwell B. Esselstyn, Jr., M.D. – heartattackproof.com
Rip Esselstyn – engine2diet.com
Matt Frazier – nomeatathlete.com
Kathy Freston – kathyfreston.com
Lauren Goebel – livelikelu.wordpress.com
Edward Goins – totalexhaustionfitness.com
Julieanna Hever – plantbaseddietitian.com
Melissa Hauser – blogger.com/profile/01241410816809750169
Attila Hildmann – attilahildmann.com
JoJo Hulett – facebook.com/VeganFitJojo
Karina Inkster – karinainkster.com
Tricia Kelly – beyondfitaustin.com/tricia-kelly.html

Tobias Klingl – facebook.com/tobias.klingl.56

Elizabeth Kucinich – facebook.com/elizabeth.kucinich

Elena Kulakovska – kulhealthyyou.com

Georges Laraque – georgeslaraque.com

Whitney Lauritsen – ecovegangal.com

Aaron MacNeil – facebook.com/groups/macneilcustomfirness

Giacomo Marchese – veganproteins.com

Dan Molls – si.com/nfl/player/dan-molls

Victoria Moran – mainstreetvegan.net

Daniel Negreanu – danielnegreanu.com

Ryan Nelson – alphafitnessmn.com

Jennifer Nicol – lifestylepuravida.com

Karen Oxley – veganbodybuilding.com

Monica Parodi – monicaparodi.com

John Pierre – johnpierre.com

Elana Priesman – plantsformation.com

Marzia Prince – MarziaPrince.com

Ani Phyo – aniphyo.com

Rich Roll – richroll.com

Joel Rosario – facebook.com/NotYourAverageVegan

Melissa Schwartz – VgirlsVguys.net

Paul Shapiro – humanesociety.org/about/leadership/executive_staff/
paul_shapiro.html

Roger Smith – facebook.com/groups/TeamVeganRhinos

Amber Sperling – facebook.com/herbivorewellness

Korin Sutton – facebook.com/korin.sutton

Thomas Tadlock – thomastadlock.com

Dani Taylor – veganproteins.com

Marcella Torres – veganmuscleandfitness.com

Derek Tresize – veganmuscleandfitness.com

Will Tucker – fitnessbywill.com

Torre Washington – thavegandread.com

Brian Wendel – forksoverknives.com

Marisa Miller Wolfson – getvegucated.com

Alicia Ziegler – facebook.com/ActressZiegler

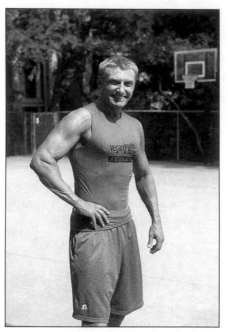

Photo by Brenda Carey

About the Author

Robert grew up on a farm in Corvallis, OR where he adopted a vegan life-style in 1995 at age 15. Today he is a best-selling author of the book *Vegan Bodybuilding & Fitness - The Complete Guide to Building Your Body on a Plant-Based Diet.*

As a two-time natural bodybuilding champion, Robert is considered one of VegNews magazine's Most Influential Vegan Athletes. He tours around the world giving talks about his story transforming from a skinny farm kid to champion vegan bodybuilder.

Robert is the founder and president of Vegan Bodybuilding & Fitness. He writes books, gives lectures around the world, and maintains the popular website, VeganBodybuilding.com. He is a regular contributor to *Vegan Health & Fitness Magazine*, a multi-sport athlete, and has followed a plant-based diet for 20 years.

For more information about Robert please visit www.veganbodybuilding. com. Robert can be reached directly by emailing info@veganbodybuilding. com, and can be found on Facebook and Twitter.